EAT
MOVE
THINK

The Path to a Healthier,
Stronger, Happier You

SHAUN FRANCIS

PUBLISHED BY SIMON & SCHUSTER

New York London Toronto Sydney New Delhi

SIMON &
SCHUSTER
CANADA

Simon & Schuster Canada
A Division of Simon & Schuster, Inc.
166 King Street East, Suite 300
Toronto, Ontario M5A 1J3

Copyright © 2018 by Medcan Health Management Inc.

This Simon & Schuster Canada edition May 2018

SIMON & SCHUSTER CANADA and colophon are
trademarks of Simon & Schuster, Inc.

For information about special discounts for bulk purchases,
please contact Simon & Schuster Special Sales at 1-800-268-3216
or CustomerService@simonandschuster.ca.

Library and Archives Canada Cataloguing in Publication
Francis, Shaun, author
Eat, move, think / Shaun Francis.
Issued in print and electronic formats.
ISBN 978-1-5011-5781-3 (hardcover).—ISBN 978-1-5011-5784-4 (ebook)
1. Health.   2. Nutrition.   3. Physical fitness.   4. Mental health.
I. Title.
RA776.F73 2018   613   C2017-906703-6
                                             C2017-907231-5

Manufactured in the United States of America

Illustrations by Damien Northmore

1   3   5   7   9   10   8   6   4   2

ISBN 978-1-5011-5781-3
ISBN 978-1-5011-5784-4 (ebook)

CONTENTS

Part Two

MOVE

Part Three

THINK

INTRODUCTION

I've worked as a CEO in the consumer health care industry for the last fifteen years. During that time, my professional and personal lives have been dominated by human wellness—how to achieve it, how to maintain it, and how to create circumstances that promote it in others. I've also spent the last decade conducting charitable work with military families. Founding Canada's True Patriot Love, the country's largest organization devoted to promoting the well-being of military families, and bringing the 2017 Invictus Games to Toronto put me into close contact with people who had made enormous sacrifices to serve their country. Over the years, I've seen some of these people demonstrate extraordinary strength as they summited mountains or cross-country skied across the polar icecap.

Our institutions, from government health bureaucracies to our military, the media we read and the experts we follow on social media, devote enormous effort to maintaining the physical health of human bodies. And that is important. But my experience with military men and women, many of whom suffer from posttraumatic stress disorder, has taught me that what's going on in our minds is just as important to achieving and maintaining wellness.

Running a health care company means constantly being asked

to make decisions on what to recommend to clients. The trouble is that, in our connected age, there's so much information available that it's difficult to distill all of that knowledge into actionable recommendations.

What complicates the task further is that medicine and the other disciplines that impact human performance—psychology, physiology, nutrition, you name it—are full of disagreements. Researchers suggest that seniors should engage in only moderate exercise roughly three times a week—unless you're one of the MDs who believe that seniors need to stress their bones with vigorous activity such as playing tennis or jumping rope. Our hearts benefit from cutting consumption of saturated fats—unless you listen to the author of a controversial study that questioned the link between saturated fat intake and heart disease. And most everyone over 70 would benefit from taking a cholesterol-lowering statin pill, say many medical professionals—except for the ones who counter that the side effects of statins may outweigh their benefits for certain people.

If you care enough about living a long, healthy, and active life to be reading this book, you may already be aware of some of these debates. You recognize that the best approach to maintaining optimum health and performance is a proactive, preventive one. So you work hard to discover new ways to get the most from yourself and your life. You educate yourself on the latest research in maintaining good health and performance. But if the experts can't agree, how can you know who to trust?

I wondered about those questions, too. Then I sought the answers to them.

I'm not a doctor or a research scientist, though. I'm a businessman, one who's always trying to find ways to be a better father, husband, and person.

I've spoken with many of the doctors and scientists who conduct research into these issues. Some of them work for one of the wellness companies I help to run—Canada's Medcan, where I'm the CEO, and EHE, an American company based in New York. Some of them use one of those companies to help them live well, for life. And still others are inspirational people I've met through charitable work.

Over the years, I've explored successful living with astronauts and Navy SEALs, Olympic champion athletes and particle physicists. "How do you maintain your edge?" I ask them. Their answers reflect the way disparate areas of life—health, job performance, physical fitness, and mental acuity—tie together.

What I learned changed my life, and my hope is that it will change yours, as well. Of course, you have to consult your health professional about tailoring any general wellness advice to your specific needs. But every person has the potential to transform our health and our life.

One approach I came across provides a neat framework for how each of us can best think about this idea of complete, well-rounded health. It came from Dr. Michael Parkinson, an MD, retired colonel in the US Air Force, and former president of the American College of Preventive Medicine.

"Eat, move, and think," he told me. "What I eat, how I move, and what I think are the greatest determinants of how long and how well we live."

I like Dr. Parkinson's approach because of its simplicity. Everybody has lots of demands on his or her time. Each of us needs to focus on the areas of our life where our effort will make the most difference to our wellness.

That's where those three ideas—*eat, move,* and *think*—come in.

To me, Dr. Parkinson nailed the three most important factors in maintaining a healthy lifestyle: diet and nutrition (eat), physical activity (move), and mental health (think).

Recently I asked my teams at Medcan and EHE to set out on a research effort to determine precisely how we can realize these ideas. We spoke to the world's experts. When they contradicted one another, we gathered together teams and distilled the research into a cohesive set of easy-to-understand pillars to health:

EAT WELL

We don't buy into fads or single-nutrient diets. Instead, we believe that arming you with knowledge will assist you to make better food choices. The best diet involves eating wholesome, minimally processed foods, mostly plant based, in reasonable quantities.

MOVE WELL

The decision to engage in regular physical activity is the most important lifestyle change you can make to increase your likelihood of living a long and active life. The best training plan involves a personalized mix of strength training, cardio, and flexibility training—with specific fitness goals and actionable plans to achieve them.

THINK WELL

Your brain is the most powerful tool you have. A fit mind is exercised regularly, using tactics such as positive self-talk, focus, visualization, proper sleep hygiene, and mindfulness.

• • •

These are the general precepts that can guide all of us to long and healthy lives. In the book that follows, I've used my own experience and the guidance of the world's experts to tackle some of the most important questions in these three all-important areas: eat, move, and think. We all want to live well and live long. Here's a road map for the journey ahead.

Part One

EAT

WHAT'S THE BEST DIET?

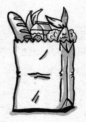

How about no diet at all? Research has shown that people aren't able to sustain most diets over the long term. That's especially true for the strict, single-nutrient-based diets that have become so popular in the last few decades, whether they're based on low fat, low carb, or high protein intake. In fact, such plans open the door to possibly harmful unintended consequences.

How many people who were following the Atkins diet in the 1990s continue to do so today? What about those who, a few years back, opted to go gluten free for reasons besides celiac disease? Rather than demonizing or lauding any single food group, we're much better off enjoying a wide variety of whole and minimally processed foods. But if you're the type of person who absolutely needs a food plan to provide you with direction on making healthier food choices, I'd suggest using one of three protocols that are almost like antidiets: the Mediterranean diet, the DASH diet, or a melding of the two approaches that encourages eaters to employ something called a MIND score.

Most diets focus on pounds lost, rather than the development of healthy eating strategies. The dieter devotes all his or her energies to following the plan, and then one of two things happens: the dieter meets the goal, returns to previous eating patterns, and gains the weight back; or the dieter gives up, feels bad about him- or herself, and gains the weight back.

Like many people, I've grappled with the difficulty of weight loss. Until my twenties, I ate whatever I wanted. That's when I graduated from the US Naval Academy and began working a desk job—and over the next decade I gained 25 pounds. The wake-up call came in my early thirties, when my primary care practitioner, Dr. Timothy Devlin, told me I needed to lose some weight. Too many soft drinks, it seemed, had caught up with me. It took me a good decade to drop the pounds required to get back to a healthy weight.

During that process, I learned that my "set point" never seemed to have increased past what it was in my early twenties. The set point is a concept used by professionals to describe the body's natural size. It explains why long-term weight loss is so difficult. If you drop too much, going far under your set point, your body uses the tactics humans evolved over millions of years to ward off starvation: it holds on to energy at a greater rate, a process known as *adaptive thermogenesis*, and deploys hormones that ramp up your hunger and delay a feeling of satiety until you've gained it all back. Basically, your body refuses to let you starve.

Nature can be cruel.

Lots of scientific studies have shown that dieting doesn't work as a weight loss strategy. In one of the most interesting ones, National Institutes of Health researchers followed up on fourteen men and women who had lost substantial amounts of weight on *The Biggest Loser*. At an average weight of 328 pounds, these people had been heavier than most at the program's beginning. They'd been provided with state-of-the-art interventions, fitness training, and weight loss techniques designed to maintain the weight loss over the long term. During the program, they'd lost an average of 129 pounds each, or 39 percent of their body weight. Six years later, the researchers found that on average they had gained back 70 percent of the weight they'd lost. More troublingly, that adaptive thermogenesis I mentioned earlier still affected the subjects, resulting in their burning 500 fewer calories per day compared to the average level for people of their weight and size. In other words, their bodies were still trying to gain back more weight.

By now we know the routine with diets. The media gloms onto a food craze, distils the message into a single phrase—gluten free, high fat, 30-day detox—and suddenly all our friends are asking the waiter to make all sorts of menu exceptions because of their latest dietary restrictions.

But many single-nutrient food fads fail to provide what they promise. Rather than promoting a healthy relationship with food in which you listen to your body, they encourage you to focus on some narrow category of food, which can lead to an inadequate mix of nutrients in your meals. Those who avoid carbohydrates, for example, leave themselves susceptible to deficiencies in fiber, folate, and thiamine.

So avoid fad diets and any single-nutrient approach. Which brings up a problem: How can you identify one? Most fad diets can be recognized by asking three questions:

DOES IT PROMISE EXTREME WEIGHT LOSS?

It doesn't matter whether you encounter the approach on a YouTube channel, in a magazine article, or in a book: if it features promotional language that promises to "melt" fat or "shed" pounds, or if it guarantees the loss of a certain amount of weight, whether that's 10, 20, or 30 pounds or even more, do yourself a favor and pass on it. Any diet that promotes itself with the promise of a steep descent in the number that stares up at you from the scale is likely a fad diet. The goal of proper nutrition should be to use what you eat as a lever to promote health and wellness—*not* to ensure that you'll look good in an outfit at a party.

DOES IT DEMONIZE AN ENTIRE SWATH OF THE GROCERY STORE?

The three macronutrients in a healthy, nutritious diet are fats, proteins, and carbohydrates. All meals should consist of a mix of all three nutrients. But that's not always the case if you follow a fad diet. The ketogenic diet says you should consume lots of fat and few carbs. The Atkins diet emphasizes protein. Neither provides the balanced mix of nutrients your body needs. Rather than artificially elevating the levels of this or that macronutrient, concentrate on enjoying a balanced diet of whole foods.

DOES IT HAVE AN EXPIRY DATE?

The 30-Day Detox, the 15-Day Cleanse, the 7-Day Reset. Wait a second: Shouldn't your approach to food be about eating well for life? Long-term good health and nutrition should be your focus. Paying attention to what you eat is a rational strategy for remaining healthy. We're trying to keep ourselves healthy for the long haul. You can't do that by crashing your weight down to an artificially low number for a short time and then going back to your old habits; there's no finish line. Instead, focus on evolving behaviors that will ensure that you make reasonable and rational food decisions for the remaining time that you're on Earth. Rather than making radical changes to your diet that will last only a few weeks, concentrate on developing healthier food behaviors that you can continue for the rest of your life.

If you come across a nutrition fad that responds "yes" to any of the above questions, you're probably better off avoiding it. Such restrictive approaches to eating can prevent you from developing the good habits that will keep you healthy for the rest of your life.

Many times a day, we make decisions to regulate what goes into our mouths and when. Those decisions impact our overall health, affecting our risk for developing everything from cancer to Alzheimer's disease, heart disease, and, of course, obesity.

We now know that fad diets aren't helpful in reaching or maintaining our health goals. In general, the best diet involves eating wholesome and minimally processed foods, mostly plant based, in reasonable quantities. But what exactly does that entail?

Here are three different strategies for eating well. None encourages strict calorie counting. None relies on an organization that will profit from your adherence to the approach. No celebrity weight loss expert advocates these diets in a transparent ploy to get you to buy his or her book. Nor are they *diets*, per se. Rather, they're dietary *patterns*—comprehensive approaches to eating well.

THE MEDITERRANEAN DIET

This is a simple approach lifted from the relationship with food employed by people in Italy, Greece, and surrounding countries. Those who follow it consume lots of fruits and vegetables, legumes, nuts, olive oil, and whole grains. They also eat fish, enjoy red wine with dinner, and tend to dine with friends and family. The eating style does not feature many foods high in saturated fats—not much red meat or butter, for example. Nor is there a lot of salt or added sugar. Researchers have conducted hundreds of studies on the effects of the dietary pattern, and found that those who follow it tend to live longer, as well as experience lower rates of heart disease, cancer, and numerous other maladies.

THE DASH DIET

An acronym for Dietary Approaches to Stop Hypertension, the DASH diet arose from a study published in 1997 that showed you can reduce blood pressure by eating lots of fruits and vegetables, legumes, nuts, low-fat dairy products, and foods that contain such blood-pressure-lowering nutrients as magnesium, potassium, and calcium. The diet was also low in saturated fat and total fat. A later DASH study showed that blood pressure could be lowered further by consuming less sodium, refined grains, and sugars. Like the Mediterranean diet, the DASH diet tends to feature higher amounts of whole grains and lower amounts of red and processed meat. Unlike the Mediterranean diet, the DASH diet includes low-fat dairy products for calcium—two to three servings per day. It's also more regimented, precisely delineating the number of servings of various food groups per week.

THE MIND DIET

Another acronym, for Mediterranean-DASH Intervention for Neurodegenerative Delay, the MIND approach is newer, based on a pair of studies published in 2015. It's basically a hybrid of the Mediterranean and DASH approaches, featuring lots of plant-based foods and limited intake of saturated fats and animal proteins. Rather than a planned-out series of meal options, the MIND approach provides a score based on how often you eat brain-healthy or brain-harmful foods. The benefits according to the research are impressive; one study found that people ranging in age from 58 to 98 who followed the approach lowered their risk of developing Alzheimer's disease— and the more closely they followed the MIND diet, the more their risk fell.

Each of these dietary approaches has its strengths and weaknesses. Those wanting to slow down cognitive decline or lower their risk of Alzheimer's disease may opt for the MIND diet; those concerned about high blood pressure may favor the DASH diet; while those who like olive oil may prefer the Mediterranean diet. Choose the one that works best for and appeals most to you—the more you like the food you're eating, the more likely you'll stick to whatever approach to eating you're following. There's a lot of information about all three available for free online, as well as numerous reference books and cookbooks available at your local bookstore. So read up and get ready to dig into a healthy, balanced diet.

À LA CARTE

Let's take a look at a meal-by-meal approach for achieving a balanced diet.

Breakfast

For me, starting the day usually involves granola or cereal and berries for breakfast. If I'm working out in the morning, I may substitute some sort of a smoothie. Whether or not you work out, eat something within an hour of waking up. It doesn't matter too much what it is, just so long as it contains approximately equal portions of protein, fiber, and fruits and vegetables. The protein promotes a feeling of fullness throughout the morning and is important for muscle and bone health, particularly among athletes. The fiber is found in foods such as oats and other whole grains. (There's also fiber in fruit.) If I'm having a smoothie, I'll throw in things such as ground flaxseed, hemp seed, or chia seed. Finally, I try to check off the "fruit and vegetable" box by eating some brightly colored berries, which have great antioxidant properties.

Morning Snack

I like a handful of almonds and maybe a small bowl of yogurt and berries. Your midmorning snack shouldn't be much—but it should be *something*, to keep up your energy level and maintain fullness through the morning.

Lunch

The midday meal should occur less than five hours after breakfast. So if you ate your first meal at 7:30, lunch at noon or even 1 p.m. works well. Half of the meal should be fruit or vegetables—a portion size of about two handfuls. A quarter of the meal, about a fist's size, should be high-quality starchy foods, whether whole grains or a starchy vegetable, such as sweet potato or butternut squash. The final quarter should be some sort of high-protein food—meat, fish, beans, or lentils.

Afternoon Snack

To keep up energy levels and ward off a midafternoon blood sugar crash, I'd encourage a snack that includes both protein and some sort of healthy carbohydrate for longer-lasting energy. Similar to the mid-morning snack, that might be a handful of nuts and a piece of fruit, such as an apple. Or it could be plain yogurt and berries or a fruit smoothie made with unsweetened soy milk.

Dinner

Dinner should be more than two hours and less than five hours from your midafternoon snack. So if your snack occurred at 4 p.m., a good time to eat dinner would be somewhere between 7 and 8 p.m. Just as with lunch, divide the plate into portions—half fruits and vegetables, a quarter whole grains or starch, and the final quarter a protein-rich food.

After Dinner

Cravings are natural. Oftentimes, they're out of your control. You've done the day, the kids are in bed, it's time for a little *you* time—and you indulge with some potato chips or a few drinks, or both. But the risk of overeating is greatest in the evening, when we're tired and our stores of discipline are low. Try to follow a policy of *dinner and done*, making a satisfying evening meal the last thing you eat for the day.

DO SATURATED FATS CAUSE CARDIOVASCULAR DISEASE?

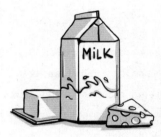

For decades, this question would have been a no-brainer—and then came the publication of a series of books and academic studies that called the conventional wisdom into question. Today the issue is surprisingly controversial—so much so that the American Heart Association took the remarkable step of issuing a presidential advisory in mid-2017. The AHA's conclusion? Eating a diet that is high in saturated fats can indeed leave you with an elevated risk of developing heart disease and stroke.

To decrease your risk of cardiovascular disease, lower your consumption of saturated fats and replace them with healthier alternatives, such as the polyunsaturated fats found in salmon, vegetable oils, and nuts and seeds or the monounsaturated fats found in olive oil and avocados.

A bit of background science here is helpful. All fats are made up of chains of carbon atoms. In saturated fats, the carbon atoms are bonded to as many hydrogen atoms as possible—that is, they're saturated with hydrogen atoms, which gives them a long, thin shape that is able to pack together tightly. That makes those fats solid at room temperature; it also means that they increase levels of "bad" cholesterol and clog the arteries. Such fats typically come from animal sources—think of butter or cheese or the fat in a steak.

The monounsaturated and polyunsaturated fats found in plants, nuts, and seeds also consist of chains of carbon atoms, but rather than all of the extra spaces on the carbon atoms bonding to hydrogen, some of them have double bonds between the carbon atoms. Those double bonds "kink" the chain, meaning that the fat molecules can't pack together tightly. Their chemical structure means that they tend to be liquid at room temperature. These fats are good for us for several reasons: they don't clog the arteries, and they can prevent and even repair the damage done by saturated fats.

In order to lower your risk of heart disease, reduce your intake of saturated fats. That doesn't mean that you should replace those calories with refined carbs and sugars. That's just replacing one bad thing with another, and it can be just as dangerous for your cardiovascular health. Instead, reduce the saturated fats in your diet and replace them with whole grains and more healthful fats, such as polyunsaturated and monounsaturated fats. Randomized controlled trials have found that replacing saturated fats with healthier unsaturated fats could reduce your risk of developing heart disease by about 30 percent—about the same effect as taking a statin.

That's a remarkable statistic. Reducing your risk of heart attack or stroke is vital for ensuring long-lasting health. Taking statins is one option, but they can cause side effects. Purely by changing the food that we put into our mouths, we can improve our health to the same extent as a powerful drug does.

You don't need to go to extremes. A teaspoon or two of butter in the course of a day is not going to give anyone a heart attack. What will elevate the risk of heart disease is a diet full of processed meats and deep-fried foods—sausage, bacon, hamburgers, French fries, and chicken fingers. The saturated fats they contain will elevate your "bad" cholesterol level, increasing your risk of developing cardiovascular disease. Instead, eat as many whole and minimally processed foods as possible.

"We can't just focus on saturated fat or sugar," says Leslie Beck, Medcan's director of food and nutrition. "You have to look at the whole diet. It isn't *just* about sugar, or *just* about saturated fats. Prefer vegetable oils to solid fats. Eat fresh fruits and vegetables, and avocados, nuts and seeds."

For those who do like to be specific, the American Heart Association suggests that those who suffer from high cholesterol limit their intake of saturated fats to 5 to 6 percent of their daily calories. Those at normal risk of developing cardiovascular disease should try to reduce their saturated fat intake below 10 percent.

To do that, try following a Mediterranean diet. Dr. Beth Abramson, Medcan's director of cardiology, acknowledges that that can be tough to do for professional people who are used to dashing to a restaurant to pick up a quick lunch that they eat at their desks. Chain restaurant meals tend to feature a lot of saturated fat and sodium.

"There are hidden fats and calories in the food we eat," she says. "So try preparing your lunch before work, at home, and take it in with you. If you're a businesswoman who eats at a restaurant seven times a week, try to reduce that to three. And when you're cooking at home, don't fry things. Bake them or grill them."

WHAT IS PROCESSED FOOD,
AND WHY IS IT SO BAD?

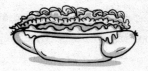

When most people say "processed food," they mean the type of packaged meals and snacks that are found at most major grocery stores. We're talking everything from potato chips to chocolate chip cookies, microwave dinners to breakfast sausages. That sort of food is denigrated by dietitians—as well as anyone who knows much about the connection between nutrition and health—because food manufacturers tend to add a lot of unnecessary sugar, salt, and fats to the snacks and meals they sell. The added ingredients make the food taste better—but they also make it much less healthful. Whenever possible, you should avoid eating highly processed foods.

That said, there are some types of processed foods that are completely fine to eat. After all, "processed" simply means that something has been done to the food in question.

For example, says Leslie Beck, Medcan's director of food and nutrition, "the frozen blueberries in my freezer have been processed"—and they're just fine to eat. "I prefer the term *ultraprocessed* foods to differentiate between the healthy and unhealthy kinds of food processing."

In other words, there's a spectrum. At one end are the things that have been altered to keep the good stuff in food. Canned fruit that is preserved in its own juices, carrot sticks, frozen broccoli, and roasted nuts—these are lightly processed foods that are fine to eat when a fresh alternative is not available. They're good options if you're pressed for time or want a bit of variety in your diet.

It's when you start getting into the premade stuff, manufactured foods that have been cooked or otherwise prepared, that you start to get into trouble. Pasta sauces and other condiments. Crackers, potato chips, and snack foods. White bread, granola bars, and refined breakfast cereals. The most highly processed foods tend to be prepared meals: frozen pizza or breaded chicken nuggets, frozen waffles, or ready-in-minutes rice or pasta dishes that can be microwaved, baked, or deep-fried. The less the food resembles its original state, the more you should avoid it.

That said, much of this stuff has become better for us as we become more educated about the food we eat, demanding healthier products for our dollars. For example, a lot of processed food was once crammed with an additive called artificial trans fat, which tended to be listed on ingredient labels as "partially hydrogenated oil." Trans fat is, like other fats, a chain of carbon atoms to which hydrogen has bonded. But trans fats are created through a chemical process called partial hydrogenation that adds hydrogen atoms into chains of naturally liquid vegetable oils. The process straightens out the fat chain, meaning the formerly liquid vegetable oil becomes, at room temperature, a solid fat. That was great for manufacturers because products that contained solid trans fats stayed fresh for longer and were easier to ship.

The problem was, trans fats turned out to be alarmingly dangerous. Studies showed that these industrially produced fats elevate levels of "bad" LDL cholesterol and decrease levels of "good" HDL cholesterol. They increase inflammatory markers and can play a role in lower birth weights in babies, obesity, type 2 diabetes, and male reproductive health. Trans fats, when compared on a gram-for-gram basis with saturated fats, elevate the risk of coronary artery disease by fifteen times.

Beginning in 2006, the US Food and Drug Administration began requiring the food industry to disclose the trans fat content in its products. Denmark was a lot more aggressive. That country's ban of trans fats in 2004 is credited with playing an important role in a 60 percent decrease in the incidence of cardiovascular disease. One study concluded that the ban had saved 14.2 lives annually per 100,000 people. The United States and Canada were slower to act. In 2015, the FDA moved to ban trans fats from American plates by 2018. The Canadian ban will take effect on September 1, 2018.

Another example of processed foods promoted with possibly misleading health-related marketing is granola bars. Many brands market themselves as health food because they contain fiber, which is tied to a lower risk of heart disease. If you look at the ingredients on many granola bars, though, the type of fiber in them is inulin, an ingredient that's isolated from chicory root. Inulin might be a fiber, but isolated fibers may not have the same benefits as the intact fibers in whole-grain foods. So you're better off passing on the granola bar and eating fruit and a handful of nuts instead.

Remember that spectrum of processing I mentioned at the beginning of this answer? Less processed food tends to be better than more processed. Making your pasta sauce from whole ingredients you've purchased yourself is better than using a jar of premade store-bought sauce. To ensure you know what you're eating, opt as much as possible for whole foods—basic ingredients such as apples, tomatoes, onions, that sort of thing. Prepare meals at home rather than relying on restaurants or fast food. Snack on whole fruits, such as apples or oranges, or on nuts. The old advice to fill most of your shopping cart with items found around the perimeter of the grocery store remains valid.

4

HOW MUCH MEAT SHOULD I EAT?

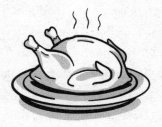

In recent years, we've all gone a little crazy for protein. Protein shakes. Protein bars. High-protein pretzels are a thing, as are high-protein breakfast cereals. Someone has even decided that cow's milk doesn't have enough protein, so they've come up with an alternative that doesn't actually contain milk but does contain 25 grams of protein in every bottle. In fact, in 2016, Americans consumed $3.8 billion worth of food products that claimed to be "an excellent source of protein"—an increase of 11.6 percent over the previous year.

Is all of this protein consumption good for our health?

First, some context. The mania for the stuff began because protein is an important macronutrient required by the body for all sorts of important functions, from building healthy bones and muscles to creating skin, nails, and hair, as well as providing enzymes and hormones.

Many people find consuming meat to be the easiest way to get their protein. But meat comes with some drawbacks. It is expensive, particularly if you're opting for the organic variety. Eating a lot of red meat is also associated with a higher risk of developing cardiovascular disease and colorectal cancer. Red meat extracts a steep environmental cost from the earth compared with vegetables. And then there are the animal cruelty issues that can make people become vegetarians or vegans.

Current dietary guidelines in the United States and Canada suggest that most sedentary people require 0.8 gram of protein per kilogram (2.2 pounds) of body mass per day, which amounts to 65 grams per day for a 180-pound man and 51 grams per day for a 140-pound woman. Frequent exercisers should get more than that, with about 1.2 grams per kilogram of body mass a good amount for the average active adult. And athletes in training who are looking to build muscle should get from 1.2 grams up to 2.0 grams per kilogram of body mass. Finally, people over the age of 65 who are looking to ward off declines in muscle tissue should try to get 1.2 grams of protein per kilogram of body mass per day.

That doesn't mean that everyone needs to run out and start gobbling up more protein than ever. People in industrialized countries such as the United States and Canada tend to get more protein than they need. For example, the average American adult male gets about 102 grams of protein per day, much more than the 56 grams his body needs. The surplus arises because people in Westernized countries often eat remarkable amounts of meat. According to a 2011 National Cancer Institute study, meat consumption in the United States is more than three times the global average. The average American consumes about 128 grams of meat per day, with 58 percent of that coming from red meat.

Make an effort to derive more protein from plant-based sources, such as beans, lentils, and tofu. Moving to diets that include higher amounts of plant-based food could have enormous health impacts, suggests a 2016 study out of Oxford University's Martin Programme on the Future of Food. The study used mathematical models to examine the impact of several scenarios. It found that if everyone in the world pursued a relatively permissive form of vegetarianism— one that also allowed the consumption of dairy products and eggs—by 2050, 7.3 million deaths could be avoided annually and 114 million life-years would be saved. The health benefits would be even greater for a vegan, or completely plant-based, diet.

Then there's the environmental issue. Producing beef, pork, and lamb creates greenhouse gases at a rate 250 times greater than production of legumes because meat is so inefficient to produce. Depending on how and where the meat is produced, the production of a single kilogram of consumed red meat creates a carbon footprint of 27 kilograms (60 pounds) of greenhouse gases, according to the Environmental Working Group. Food-related greenhouse gas could amount to more than half the world's emissions by 2050, according to the Oxford study.

If everyone went vegetarian, food-related emissions worldwide could decrease by 63 percent. Going without red meat and getting your protein from such sources as chicken, fish, or eggs for just one day per week for a year is the equivalent of not driving 760 miles, according to a 2008 study from Carnegie Mellon University. And if you opted on that single day each week to get your protein exclusively from plant-based sources? That would be the equivalent of not driving 1,160 miles.

All that said, I'm not a vegetarian, nor are most of the registered dietitians on my nutrition team. Part of the reason, for me, at least, is that I think meat tastes good—and we should enjoy our food. A good rule for meat consumption is that a serving of meat should never amount to more than a quarter of your plate. Another way to think of it is that your meat portion should never be larger in size or thicker than your palm.

But what *kind* of meat is best? My people come from Stellarton, Nova Scotia, where the coal miners ate as much steak as they could afford. Red meats such as steak do have some benefits. On top of containing such nutrients as niacin, riboflavin, and other B vitamins, red meat is a source of iron, which is good for the body because it helps the blood transport oxygen. It takes some work to get enough iron if you're not eating red meat. So feel free to eat red meat, but limit yourself to two or three times a week.

There isn't much of a ceiling for chicken and fish. Feel free to eat those as frequently as you like, but keep in mind that deriving protein from a variety of foods, including plant-based sources, will benefit the body most. Try for three servings of fish a week. Fish is good for your health because it's a great source of omega-3 fats and is low in saturated fats. Consuming up to two 3-ounce servings of fatty fish—such as salmon, mackerel, sardines, or herring—each week has been shown to decrease the risk of dying by heart disease by 36 percent. That said, be sure to avoid types of fish known to contain high levels of mercury, such as shark, king mackerel, and golden snapper.

Great plant-based sources of protein include such foods as soybeans, chickpeas, lentils, nuts, and seeds. You can start by trying to go three to four meals without meat—or perhaps try going without it on a "meatless Monday" or any other day of the week. My team and I have seen this work many times over. Most people don't notice that they've done without meat, and they're eating more healthfully at the same time.

In general try to consume protein at most meals to feel full, prevent cravings, and maintain your muscle mass. But for personal health and environmental sustainability, try to incorporate plant-based protein sources such as soybeans, legumes, whole grains, seeds, and nuts into your diet. Limit your red meat consumption to a serving the size and thickness of your palm, two or three times a week, and try to eat fatty fish and seafood two or three times a week because they're a great source of omega-3 fatty acids.

5

WHAT IF I WANT TO LOSE WEIGHT AND STILL KEEP MY MUSCLE MASS?

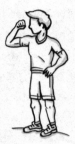

We all have in our head an idea of weight loss that sees body fat melt away, leaving behind a chiseled physique of abdominals, biceps, and glutes. But research has found that, all things being equal, about 25 percent of any weight you lose is muscle.

That's a problem for athletes who are trying to retain as much lean muscle mass as possible. I have confronted this myself. I'm an avid cyclist who has experienced some of the best moments of my life while cruising quiet country roads on two wheels. Weight is important to cyclists, because every extra ounce is more mass that has to be propelled forward. Some people pay thousands of dollars to buy components that shave a few ounces off a road bike. Another way to improve one's average speed on a ride is to shave some weight from the human body in the saddle. Ideally, you want to do that without losing any muscle. Similar efforts are made in many other forms of athletics, from rowing, swimming, and running to hockey, soccer, and mixed martial arts.

Luckily, science has discovered a method that allows the reten-tion, and even the gain, of muscle mass while losing weight. The worldwide expert on this process is Stuart Phillips, who runs the Exercise Metabolism Research Group at McMaster University.

Phillips points out that protein is a peculiarly tricky macronutri-ent for the body to manage because we don't have the capability of storing it. It's not like fat; when we eat food that contains protein, the body's digestive system processes it, whisks it into our blood-stream, and transports it throughout the body, where some of it is used to produce muscle and bone. Then, some hours after we've eaten, when all the protein has been distributed, the process stops—until we eat again.

Phillips has conducted numerous experiments to determine the best configuration of protein dosing to help the body create as much muscle as possible during training. The answer he came up with is 0.25 gram of protein per kilogram of body weight per meal or 0.11 gram of protein per pound of body weight.

One thing to remember here is that his research was based on meals that took place every four hours. So his test subjects might have eaten at 6 a.m., 10 a.m., 2 p.m., and 6 p.m. On top of that, the subjects consumed a *double* dose of protein at 10 p.m., immediately before bed.

Let's say you're a 220-pound man engaged in resistance train-ing. To ensure that your body has the protein it needs to build as much muscle as it can, Phillips's studies suggest that you should be consuming around 25 grams of protein every four hours, plus that 50-gram double dose before bed, for a total of 150 grams of protein per day. A 130-pound woman looking to provide her body with enough protein to maximally build muscle should be consuming 15 grams of protein at the same intervals.

But what if you're looking to lose weight—as cyclists like me might want to do before a big race? Remember how 25 percent of the pounds you lose amount to lost muscle? Essentially, Phillips was trying to see whether he could change that. He took forty young overweight university-aged men and required them to go through a remarkably tough training regimen. Of that group, twenty ate a low-calorie, high-protein diet—up to 2.4 grams per kilogram of body weight per day, for a total of 240 grams of protein a day. (That's a lot of protein—your typical 4-ounce boneless, skinless chicken breast has about 25 grams of protein.) The others ate a normal diet.

WHAT DOES 25 GRAMS OF PROTEIN LOOK LIKE?

These are just for reference's sake—I'm not suggesting you eat a cup of flaxseed meal in one sitting. Also, bear in mind that the nutrient content of food varies depending on what you're eating. Check the label if precision is your aim.

4 ounces of turkey, pork, or chicken (about the size of a deck of cards)

4 ounces of steak

4-ounce patty of cooked ground beef

1 cup of ground flaxseed meal

5 cups of cooked brown long-grain rice

9 tablespoons of uncooked black beans

9 tablespoons of raw tofu

1 cup of Greek yogurt

1 cup of low-fat cottage cheese

3 cups of 2 percent milk

7 tablespoons of smooth peanut butter

4 large eggs

1 cup of shredded mozzarella cheese

1⅓ cups of cooked lentils

1 cup of dry steel-cut oats

3 cups of cooked quinoa

1 cup of whole almonds

Phillips wanted to see whether the high-protein, low-calorie diet would help prevent losing muscle mass. It did. In fact, at the end of the month, the men in the test group had actually *gained* lean body mass. They were also radically stronger and faster. Their maximum bench press weight went up by 86 pounds, their maximum leg press weight doubled, and they dropped three and a half minutes from their cycling time trial. More than that, they lost an average of 10.5 pounds of fat and gained about 2.5 pounds of muscle mass.

Phillips had succeeded in changing the usual way human bodies lose weight—and had done so by giving his test subjects the maximal amount of protein their bodies could use.

Research like Phillips's helps to explain the rise of high-protein snacks of all sorts. It's pretty hard to get that much protein from normal food. Can you imagine eating eight boneless, skinless chicken breasts *every day*? Once they're tired of chicken and meats, a lot of people turn to supplements, such as protein bars and protein powder.

Protein powders are fine—as long as you consume them as just one option among many and don't rely exclusively on them to replace meals on a regular basis.

There are two reasons to be wary of relying too heavily on

protein supplements. First, proteins consist of amino acids, and the body requires numerous different types of amino acids. The particular protein supplement you're using may not provide you with all the amino acids you need. Consequently, it's important to get your protein from a variety of food sources to ensure that you're getting all the essential amino acids.

Second, many protein powders and bars are sweetened with added sugars and include additives or preservatives. Try to ensure that the protein powder you're using doesn't contain any added sugar. Whey protein, derived from cow's milk, is considered the best sort of protein powder because it contains a higher amount of essential amino acids—the ones the body can't make on its own. The quality of whey protein powders can vary, and numerous brands exist. Choose one that has at least 90 percent protein content, which can be easily calculated by dividing the protein content listed on the ingredients label by the serving size.

6

HOW CAN I QUIT WORRYING ABOUT MY WEIGHT AND CONCENTRATE ON GETTING HEALTHY?

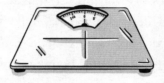

Dieting and traditional approaches to weight loss just don't work for some people, especially those who have to manage complicating factors such as genetic conditions, injuries, and predisposition to certain illnesses. If that's the case for you, you may benefit from a completely different path—one that removes the emphasis from weight loss altogether. That's the approach advocated by the American writer and physiology PhD Linda Bacon.

Over the last decade or so, Bacon has become the best-known proponent of the Health at Every Size (HAES) movement, which preaches an acceptance of our bodies, no matter the number that shows on the scale. The energy that HAES followers once devoted to losing weight is instead channeled into developing a healthy body image, exercising for the enjoyment of the activity, and monitoring the body's appetite and eating cues. And here's the encouraging thing—it turns out that some people who stop focusing on their weight and concentrate on getting healthy actually end up losing weight in the process.

It's an unconventional notion for many members of the health care community, particularly because the evidence suggests that the so-called obesity epidemic is growing worse around the globe. One of the largest-ever studies of its kind, published in July 2017 in *The New England Journal of Medicine* and using data from 195 countries, concluded that "the prevalence of obesity has more than doubled since 1980 and is now 5% in children and 12% in adults," according to an accompanying editorial.

Those stats are global. Prevalence rates in Canada and the United States are much higher, with about a quarter of Canadian adults qualifying as obese.

The study did have some positive news, though. The high body mass index (BMI) levels don't seem to be increasing death and disability rates. In fact, developing research shows that being overweight or even mildly obese may be less risky than we once thought. One much-cited 2013 paper in *The Journal of the American Medical Association* found that overweight people—classified as having a BMI between 25 and 29.9 kg/m^2—actually had a lower risk of mortality than normal-weight people.

The findings have contributed to a new idea that there isn't a single "ideal" weight, that each individual's healthy weight range could be different, and that each of us should focus more on getting healthy than on losing weight. That thinking has only become more popular, thanks to the Health at Every Size program and others like it.

"We see people all the time who are so obsessed with getting their weight to an arbitrary number," says Stefania Palmeri, a registered dietitian at Medcan. Palmeri says this militancy doesn't make sense from a health perspective. "It can drive an unhealthy fixation on food rules which, too often, undermines overall nutrition. And we need to remember that weight is just one factor among many when it comes to health."

Plenty of obese people try hard to lose weight. But sometimes our bodies work against us. For example, if the body has a significant caloric deficit—that is, if it takes in considerably fewer calories than it needs to maintain its weight—its metabolic rate slows. This process, known as metabolic adaptation, works against weight loss goals.

Health at Every Size suggests that rather than obsessing about your weight, you try listening to your body's cues of appetite and fullness. Transfer the energy once devoted to trying to lose weight into developing a healthy relationship with food, higher self-esteem, and exercising for the joy of it.

"We have to look at all the messages food can give us," Bacon says. The challenge is noticing those messages; for example, that the high that comes from the sugar in fruit lasts longer than that which comes from the added sugar in junk food, because the fruit contains fiber and a high-fiber diet makes you feel better. Or take chocolate. The first couple of bites of chocolate taste great. But then there's less and less of a taste response. The fourth and fifth bites of chocolate don't taste as good as the first ones; someone who is paying attention to food signals might interpret that as a message to put the chocolate aside. Over time, we can learn that eating smaller amounts of food is a way to maximally derive enjoyment from it; quality over quantity, as it were.

Many people apply to Bacon and other followers of the HAES philosophy, asking to lose weight. When that happens, Bacon asks people to step back and examine what they're looking to get out of their weight loss. "We're not saying you will lose weight, we're not saying you won't," she says. "What we *are* saying is, you won't fight your body anymore. You'll feel good about the choices you're making. That's liberating."

Another benefit? The approach can encourage people to take up exercise. "Many people have been taught exercise is their punishment for eating too much or weighing too much," Bacon says. "When exercise has been pitched as something you're supposed to do, it's hard to make that a sustainable practice. We call it a *work*out. That doesn't sound like fun. It's like a medical prescription as opposed to something that makes you feel good. But when exercise is the reward, it's fun, it's what they look forward to, and it naturally becomes a part of their lives. That's a helpful change of frame for people."

So if you're feeling frustrated with a long-term inability to lose weight, consider shifting your focus from the numbers on your scale toward more productive efforts, such as getting healthy and developing a better relationship with food. The results might surprise you.

7

HOW MUCH COFFEE SHOULD I DRINK?

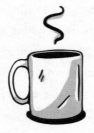

My physicians get this question a lot. It's something I used to wonder, too, particularly after I underwent genetic testing and discovered that my DNA means that I metabolize coffee more slowly than average. Research reveals that the "sweet spot" for coffee consumption is somewhere between three and five cups per day.

That's a lot different from the old recommendation. It used to be that health authorities made people feel guilty about their coffee consumption. For example, a panel of experts convened by the World Health Organization to study the issue back in 1991 placed coffee in the same category as lead and diesel fuel, rated "possibly carcinogenic." In particular, coffee consumption was thought to be associated with bladder and pancreatic cancer.

That troubled me, because I like my coffee. I'll usually have three or four cups a day. It wakes me up in the morning and perks me up before a midafternoon meeting. And plenty of people out there are just like me.

Luckily, scientists continued to conduct research into the link between coffee and overall mortality. One breakthrough came when they found a flaw in the old studies: coffee drinkers tend to smoke at higher rates than the general population, and the increased smoking may have accounted for the increased cancer risk. When they figured out how to isolate the results of coffee drinking from those of smoking, they discovered that coffee drinking was actually associated with *decreased* rates of cancer, as well as some other maladies.

Dr. Frank Hu at the Harvard T.H. Chan School of Public Health looked into those data. He tracked the coffee-drinking patterns of more than 200,000 male and female health professionals over thirty years, then compared them with the mortality data of the same group.

Hu's study found that people who drank three to five cups of coffee per day were at a lower risk of premature death from certain illnesses than to those who didn't drink coffee or drank only a small amount each day. It didn't matter whether the coffee was caffeinated or decaffeinated—moderate coffee drinking decreased the risk of death from such maladies as cardiovascular disease, diabetes, depression and suicide, liver disease, and even neurodegenerative diseases such as Parkinson's disease.

The evidence is so compelling that the same WHO group that concluded that coffee may be "possibly carcinogenic" has recategorized the beverage. The group concluded that coffee actually cuts the risk of developing uterine and liver cancer. It turns out that coffee creates strong antioxidant benefits in the body. Swirling around in it are such anti-inflammatories as magnesium, chlorogenic acid, lignans, and quinides.

Granted, not everyone is going to want to drink three to five cups of *caffeinated* coffee a day. Too much caffeine can affect stress levels. Nor are large amounts recommended for those with hypertension. US and Canadian guidelines suggest limiting caffeine consumption to 300 milligrams a day for women of childbearing age and 400 milligrams a day for other healthy adults. Those with hypertension may want to limit their consumption to 200 milligrams a day.

That 400 milligrams is equivalent to about four cups of coffee, if your mug contains 8 fluid ounces or 250 milliliters. For reference, a grande Americano from Starbucks has 225 milligrams of caffeine, while a medium brewed coffee from Tim Hortons contains 205 milligrams.

CAFFEINE-CRAZED

Here's the caffeine content of a few of the more popular drinks.

Red Bull energy drink, 8-ounce or 250 ml can: 80 mg

Monster Energy drink, 16 ounces or 473 ml: 160 mg

Starbucks caffè mocha, grande size: 175 mg

Lipton Tea, 6 ounces or 180 ml, five-minute steep time: 43 mg

Coca Cola, 12-ounce or 355 ml can: 34 mg

Mountain Dew, 12-ounce or 355 ml can: 55 mg

Average home-brewed 8-ounce or 250 ml cup of coffee: 95 mg

Luckily, decaffeinated coffee will provide you with most of the life-extending benefits of the caffeinated variety. To balance the health benefits of coffee with your need for caffeine, try switching to decaf after the third or fourth cup of the day.

Another good practice is to avoid adding sugar to your coffee. A woman who adds two teaspoons of sugar to each cup of coffee she drinks will reach her maximum daily sugar intake on her third cup.

It takes only a week or two to learn to like coffee without any added sugar. Last, the Hu study noted that coffee drinkers who smoked did not experience the same benefits from the brewed drink. So don't smoke—and tomorrow morning, perhaps you can enjoy your coffee without any guilt.

8

CAN WHAT I EAT AFFECT
MY MENTAL HEALTH?

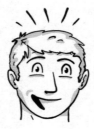

The answer is an unadulterated "yes." What we put into our mouths affects what happens in our brains on a number of different levels and in numerous different ways. In the short term, alcohol can dull the brain, and not eating enough can make us irritable. Over the long term, a poor diet can leave us susceptible to mental health issues such as depression.

One of my associates told me about a great sign that hangs in a restaurant in the vacation town of Southampton, Ontario: "I'm sorry about what I said when I was hungry." I've had to say an apology like this to my wife on occasion. It's something that I've experienced on longer cycling sessions, too; particularly if I've really been cranking on the pedals, I'll notice that negativity can start to invade my stream of consciousness. When I hear that negative voice in the back of my head, I'll reach into my jersey pocket for an energy bar, and mere seconds after I've started chewing, I'll find that I'm miraculously feeling more positive about everything—even the next hill climb.

The link between diet and mental health isn't studied as much as it should be. That may have something to do with the way people in the developed world think about mind and body—as two separate entities, insulated from each other. Keeping biology apart from psychology is a convention we use to convince ourselves how enlightened we are. The body is biology and nature and animal. What separates us from the rest of nature happens in the mind: the brain and psychology.

In reality, that's nonsense. The body affects what's going on in the brain every minute of every day. It starts in the morning, when we use the caffeine in coffee to perk ourselves up. Breakfast provides essential nutrients to the blood, which in turn gets them into the cells. And if we don't eat enough, we get that "hangry" effect referenced in the apology sign.

Diet can also affect our mental health in more significant ways. I first grasped just how neglected this aspect of human health is when I came across an article about a Columbia University psychiatrist, Dr. Drew Ramsey, who had compiled a list of "brain-essential nutrients." According to Dr. Ramsey, eating foods rich in these nutrients decreases the incidence of depression and improves the treatment of depression in those already afflicted with the disease.

Clinical psychologists such as the New York–based Dr. Michael Friedman agree with Dr. Ramsey. When someone seeks treatment for depression, we tend to treat the condition with medical or psychological tools—antidepressant drugs, perhaps, or talk therapy. Friedman believes that lifestyle issues, such as poor nutrition and eating habits, can play a causal role in the onset of depression. Following that line of thinking, he believes that clinicians who treat depression need to look into dietary causes before they move on to biological or psychological therapies.

DR. RAMSEY'S BRAIN-ESSENTIAL NUTRIENTS

Long-chain omega-3 fatty acids

Magnesium

Calcium

Fiber

B vitamins, especially thiamine, folate, and B12

Vitamins D and E

"When I work with someone," says Friedman, who has a PhD in psychology from Yale University, "before I even start talking about what their issues are, we have to get them eating healthy, exercising, sleeping well."

Friedman first started noticing the link between physical and mental health when dealing with binge eaters. "One of the main treatments of binge eating is having a regular, structured diet. A lot of people who binge eat—they won't eat any breakfast, and they'll have a bunch of coffee because they're rushing and they're frantic and because they kind of like the idea that if they drink coffee they won't eat anything," he says. "They don't eat much through the day and then finally for dinner they have something, and *then*, for some odd reason, they wind up taking in, like, five thousand calories at night—which then leads them to not sleep. They don't exercise because they're too tired, and then they feel terrible about themselves the following morning, when they start the whole cycle all over again."

But it's not just the timing of calorie intake that plays a role in mental health. Research has found that those who follow a whole-food, plant-based diet also have lower rates of depression. Some studies have shown a 30 percent reduction in risk of depression for those who adhere to a Mediterranean diet. Similarly, studies find higher rates of depression among those who follow what's regarded as a poor diet—high in refined carbohydrates, sugars, and heavily processed foods.

An Australian study published in 2017 demonstrates just how powerful diet can be to ward off depression. The trial featured two groups of people drawn from a population suffering from major depressive episodes. One group received seven nutrition counseling sessions designed to improve the participants' eating patterns. The other group simply engaged in seven sessions of friendly conversation with trained research assistants. After twelve weeks, the diet-support group improved more than the group that didn't receive any dietary help.

The study was small. And nutrition-based research is notoriously difficult to do well. But the indications are clear: those suffering from depression, or who believe they are at risk of suffering from depression, would do well to consider how their eating patterns may be contributing to their mental health issues. An improved diet—one that's lower in unhealthy fat and highly processed foods and includes more plants and whole foods—may help a case of depression. And controlling your hunger level throughout the course of a day will certainly help keep you even-tempered.

9

SHOULD OLDER PEOPLE EAT
DIFFERENTLY FROM THE YOUNG?

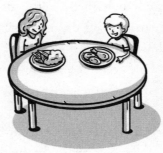

Absolutely—for a number of different reasons. The bodies of older people require fewer calories, yet their nutrient requirements stay constant or even increase. As a result, the foods that older people eat should be more nutrient dense. Following a certain kind of healthful diet also has been associated with an increased ability to ward off Alzheimer's disease and preserve cognitive function. And paying greater attention to protein intake can help to ward off the age-related decline in muscle mass.

Let's start with calories. Older people require fewer calories than the young since their resting metabolic rate—the number of calories the body burns at rest—declines by 1 to 2 percent per decade. In general, women require 7 fewer calories a day every year past 30, while men require 10 calories less per day. So a 65-year-old man needs to eat 350 fewer calories per day than he did when he was 30. I've found that my own aging has involved a steady cutting back on dietary indulgences. As a teenager and into my twenties, I could eat anything I wanted. Once I hit 30, I had to cut back on the chocolate bars and the soda—an effect not only of aging but also of the fact that I was sitting at a desk more often.

These days, I restrict my indulgent eating. But even accounting for the decrease in calories my body requires, as I transition from my middle age to my senior years I'll likely ease off and allow myself a little more indulgence.

"You kind of want to be a bear," Dr. James Aw, Medcan's chief medical officer, says. "You want to have some weight in reserve—you don't want to be *too* thin."

So as you get older, you want to have something in store for a rainy day—without tipping into obesity. "For my older patients," says Dr. Aw, "if you're eighty and healthy, and doing what you want, who am I to deny you? If you want a bar of dark chocolate every night, who am I to say you can't? Aging gracefully shouldn't be about suffering. It should be about enjoying life."

As we age, our nutrient requirements change. Protein intake becomes progressively more important, for example, to assist with muscle repair. And calcium intake becomes more important to maintain bone strength; it may also play a role in managing hypertension. Women over the age of 50 should boost their calcium intake from 1,000 milligrams a day to 1,200 milligrams. Men should do the same thing after the age of 70.

People over the age of 50 should also supplement their diets with vitamin B12, which is good for brain health. A third of people over the age of 50 don't produce enough of a protein called *gastric intrinsic factor*. The lack of this protein prevents them from absorbing enough vitamin B12 from food, which, in turn, can lead to cognitive issues. Supplementing what one gets from dietary sources provides enough of an extra dose to help prevent the problem.

MIND DOS AND DONT'S

Dos
- ✓ Green leafy vegetables
- ✓ Other vegetables (such as green or red peppers, squash, carrots, broccoli)
- ✓ Nuts
- ✓ Berries
- ✓ Beans (including lentils and soybeans)
- ✓ Whole grains
- ✓ Seafood (including tuna sandwich and any fresh fish dish, but not fried fish cakes or sticks)
- ✓ Poultry
- ✓ Olive oil
- ✓ Wine

Don'ts
- ✗ Red meats (including cheeseburgers, beef tacos, hot dogs)
- ✗ Butter and stick margarine
- ✗ Cheese
- ✗ Pastries and sweets (including milk shakes and frappés, ice cream, danishes, donuts, cakes, and sweet rolls)
- ✗ Fried/fast food (such as French fries and chicken nuggets)

Finally, and possibly most important, anyone who is concerned about preserving his or her cognitive function for as long as possible—and this goes for people of all ages—should seriously consider the MIND dietary approach. A pair of US studies demonstrated that foods such as green leafy vegetables and berries protect against declines in cognitive performance, possibly because they contain high amounts of folate, vitamin E, carotenoids, and flavonoids. So the designers of the MIND approach to eating encourage their subjects to include lots of those foods in their meals.

The pioneers of the MIND approach assessed the eating patterns of just under 1,000 elderly people over approximately five years. They also assessed the same people for cognitive function. When they compared the results, they found that high MIND scores were associated with preserved cognitive function. In fact, the people whose MIND scores were in the highest third tended to have cognitive function on a par with someone 7.5 years younger. Similarly, the subjects who fell into the highest third of MIND scores were 53 percent less likely to develop Alzheimer's disease than were the lowest-scoring third.

Many other studies have demonstrated similar effects, which underscores the important takeaway: following healthy eating habits seems to protect the brain from the effects of aging. You're never too young to adopt healthy dietary patterns—but they become doubly important when you're elderly.

10

CAN I HAVE DESSERT AFTER DINNER?

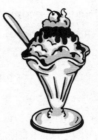

In a word, yes. But be careful about your portion size. I have a sweet tooth, and my sugar intake has been an ongoing preoccupation. To manage it, I've broken down my approach to a few easy rules. I don't drink sugar-sweetened beverages, including everything from flavored carbonated beverages to energy drinks to soft drinks such as lemonade and iced teas—anything that food manufacturers have crammed with sugar. Nor do I add sugar to my coffee. I also avoid sugary snacks during the day. If I've followed these rules, I allow myself to enjoy a modest serving of dessert after dinner.

Sugar has been demonized in the nutritional literature lately, with the playwright Paul Rudnick noting that there is a "war on sugar." "Many books and studies are asserting that sugar causes or contributes to multiple fatal illnesses, costing billions of dollars in health care each year. I dispute none of this," remarked Rudnick in the *New York Times*. "But I would like to add that sugar tastes really, really good."

I agree with Rudnick. So does science. Researchers observe that even infants demonstrate a taste for sweet things. A sweet taste tells the brain that the mouth has encountered a possible energy source. The craving increases with age at least into adolescence.

That said, in evolutionary terms we haven't been consuming the ingredient most associated with sweetness—sugar—for very long. The average American's annual consumption of sugar has increased to a startling 120 pounds, or 30 times what it was in the eighteenth century. Canadian consumption demonstrates a similar trend, as does that of most other industrialized countries. Consumption has backed off in the last twenty years, but we're still taking in too much sugar. In fact, the World Health Organization is so concerned about our consumption and the worldwide increase in obesity to which it's linked that in 2015, it recommended cutting sugar intake back to 5 percent of daily calories, which is about 25 grams a day for women following a standard 2,000-calorie diet, and 36 grams per day for men—both of which are below the 39 grams of sugar found in a *single* 12-ounce (355 ml) can of Coca-Cola.

Why so little? The WHO is worried about tooth decay—and sugar consumption is associated with numerous health problems, from tooth decay to higher risk for the development of Alzheimer's disease to faster aging. One study even linked greater consumption of sugar-sweetened beverages with lower brain volume and worse performance on memory tests. Reducing sugar has been tied to rapid improvement in biological markers of heart health. It's also thought to play a major role in the previously unknown emergence of fatty liver disease in children. It's even been tied to cancer.

That said, the war on sugar may be causing some collateral damage. "Sugar has become dietary enemy number one," observed the *Guardian* newspaper. Anytime the media demonize a single nutrient, unintentional consequences can result. For example, the demonization of fat likely played a factor in the massive uptick in sugar consumption from 1950 to 2000.

My nutrition team is seeing people take extraordinary steps to reduce their sugar consumption. Some people are even cutting out fruit because they're concerned about the sugar content in oranges or strawberries. Don't do that. "Naturally occurring sugar in fruit comes packaged with fiber that functions to slow down the absorption of sugar into the bloodstream," says Leslie Beck, Medcan director of food and nutrition.

So how to decrease your sugar consumption? Start by cutting sugar-sweetened beverages from your diet. Just don't drink them. Not ever.

THE PROBLEM OF DIET SODA

Diet soft drinks may be as problematic for your long-term health as the sugar-sweetened beverages they're supposed to replace. Something about the way the body responds to the artificial sweeteners is thought to prevent us from properly registering the intake of calories; the sweeteners hamper our ability to feel full when we should. They also may harm gut bacteria in a manner that prevents us from properly metabolizing sugar. So be careful—the diet versions of your favorite soft drinks may come with health risks all their own.

Next, quit drinking coffee with sugar. In Canada, the double double (two teaspoons of sugar and two creams) at Tim Hortons amounts to the national drink. Starbucks' Frappuccino sales form a significant slice of the company's annual sales. Both drinks are filled with granulated sugar, and one teaspoon of granulated sugar amounts to 4 grams. So a person who drinks two double double coffees by 10 a.m. has already had 16 grams of sugar—more than half the maximum suggested limit for women and close to half the limit for men.

Finally, those who are big yogurt eaters should move away from flavored products to plain versions that they flavor themselves. Fruit and vanilla yogurt flavors were originally marketed as desserts but today are regularly consumed as breakfast or snacks. Their sugar content can be shockingly high. A tiny 100-gram tub of vanilla- or fruit-flavored Greek yogurt delivers 8 grams of added sugar. Switching to plain yogurt and getting your sweetness from fruit will substantially cut your consumption of added sugar. Another trick? Sprinkle cinnamon onto plain yogurt to add flavor.

If you've done all that—avoided soda, cut sugar from your coffee, and reduced the overall added sugar in such foods as flavored yogurts—I don't see a major problem in allowing yourself a modest portion of dessert, particularly if it includes a healthful, fiber-containing fruit, such as a poached pear or grilled pineapple.

11

IS THERE ANY TRUTH TO THE
FIVE-SECOND RULE?

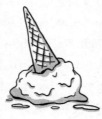

As proclaimed by youth everywhere, the five-second rule is the length of time food can safely sit on the ground before it becomes infested with too many germs to eat. Say you're a 13-year-old at a local summer festival and you've just dropped a Pogo that you earned with twenty minutes of waiting in line. "Five-second rule," you might say and swiftly reach down to rescue the junk food, perhaps dusting off a few bits of grit and dust.

I'm not aware of any scientific basis for the five-second rule. How much bacteria actually transfers to the food after the first exposure? I checked with one of the smartest clinicians I know, Dr. Tania Elliott, the chief medical officer at EHE.

"The longer something sits on the ground, the more contaminated it will become," says Dr. Elliott. "The surface also matters—bacteria is less likely to transfer right away if something is dropped on a carpet. Steel and tile, however, have a higher rate of transfer. But that isn't to say that all germs should be avoided."

It turns out that many of those germs that so concerned our

parents a generation ago are today understood to form an integral part of our biology. Countless bacteria reside on the skin, in the respiratory tract, and most of all in the gut. They aren't harmful to our health; in fact, they're necessary for the body to work properly. And they're remarkably numerous. The gut has a bacterial population of approximately 100 trillion, according to Dr. Linda Lee, the director of endoscopy at Johns Hopkins Hospital. There's about a kilogram's worth of bacteria in the colon alone.

These bacteria help the body in numerous ways. They assist with the proper digestion of food. There's some proof that they play a role in the regulation of mood and anxiety. And they help the immune system work properly by preventing unfriendly microbes from harming the body.

"We grew up during a time when we learned that bacteria are bad for us," says Dr. Lee. "But it turns out that these bacteria in our intestines are really beneficial."

That's a message that first began to transition from the academic journals to the greater populace several years back. The news has prompted certain quarters of the food industry to roll out all sorts of products designed to bolster the health of the body's bacteria—what academics refer to as our gut flora, or microbiota.

In contrast to the five-second rule, which was designed to prevent germs from getting into our bodies, food manufacturers today are creating products with the express purpose of getting *more* bacteria into our bellies.

There is some scientific basis for what they're trying to do. Bacteria do have to get into the body somehow, after all. In utero, the fetal gut is sterile. But a gut that stays sterile—that is, totally uninhabited by bacteria—would create all sorts of immune system problems for its owner.

So how do all those germs get in there? One important way is via birth. An infant gets its first supply of bacteria from its mother—when going through the birth canal and by feeding on breast milk, among other ways.

"Probably the most important determinant of the bacteria in the gut, however, is diet," says Dr. Lee. If you eat a plant-based diet, it will skew your gut microbiome in one direction. A diet heavy in red meat and fat will send your microbiome in a different direction.

So what's a healthy microbiome? According to Dr. Lee, a healthy gut is populated by a microbiome that looks a bit like downtown Manhattan or Toronto. It's crowded and diverse. In the same way that a thriving urban core benefits from lots of different ethnicities and ages, a gut benefits from lots of different types of bacteria.

"The more populated, the more diverse, and the more productive our bacterial communities are, the more beneficial they are to us as human beings," says Dr. Lee.

Problems arise, then, not when there are too many bacteria but when there are too few. Again, it's similar to the example of a city center: when residents move away from an urban core, problems such as increased crime or commuting delays can develop.

A similar phenomenon can happen in the gut. Antibiotics can wipe out the density and diversity of a gut's bacterial population. Most people's guts will return to their previous diversity in two to four weeks. But sometimes the old bacteria don't return. And in their place, less friendly elements—bad bacteria, fungi, or viruses—can take over. That can lead to numerous health concerns, such as irritable bowel syndrome, obesity, and even mental health problems.

Which brings us to probiotics. Probiotics are bacteria that are thought to be beneficial to the gut and our overall health. They can be purchased over the counter as supplements, pills, or powders. They can also be added to certain foods during the manufacturing process. Probiotics have been a frequent source of questions to my staff in recent years. The people who partner with us ask whether they should be taking probiotics. And the answer, in most cases, is: probably not.

Some types of probiotics have been shown to be beneficial for certain types of conditions. For example, Dr. Lee says that children with viral diarrhea have benefited from taking a strain of bacteria, *Lactobacillus acidophilus*, often referred to simply as acidophilus.

But probiotics aren't well regulated by health authorities in the United States. The fast-growing product segment features dozens of different bacterial strains, and researchers haven't yet fully studied the benefits of each strain. Different types of bacteria can help with different conditions. "For most consumers," says Dr. Lee, "it's hard to tell which is the right probiotic strain to take."

Another approach that's gaining currency in some circles is the suggestion to eat foods that have fermented—that have played host to bacterial reactions. Yogurt, for example, is the result of bacteria fermenting milk. Miso, sauerkraut, kimchi—each of these foods possesses a distinctive taste thanks to bacterial reactions.

Those foods might taste great, but the health benefits of the bacteria in them are still being debated. It's also important to note that the few foods whose bacterial populations have been shown to survive digestion in the human gut, such as some cured meats and cheeses, may come with their own health risks when eaten in large quantities. In the case of yogurt, it's not clear that the bacteria survive the fermentation process.

"Some food manufacturers have a tendency to want to make claims that may not actually yet be proven," remarks Dr. Lee, describing a multimillion-dollar settlement of a class action lawsuit against Dannon, a case that prompted the yogurt maker to change its claims involving the effect of its DanActive yogurt drink and Activia yogurt.

Finally, it's difficult to specify which probiotic strain may be best for which person. "What could be good for your sister could be very different for you," says Dr. Lee.

Researchers have not yet established that taking probiotics is beneficial for general health, longevity, or cancer prevention. Because so much remains unknown about probiotics and their effect on human health, Dr. Lee refrains from suggesting her patients take them. If you do wish to take a probiotic, she suggests that you follow the product's dosage guidelines for a month. Then, if the product doesn't cause the effect that you're seeking, move on to another strain—or stop taking a probiotic altogether.

Some techniques to ensure the health of your gut flora include minimizing antibiotic use and maintaining a healthy body weight. That said, there is one particularly effective dietary method that will help ensure the diversity and health of gut flora: eat a high-fiber diet. Foods such as oats, lentils, split peas, and lima beans provide fuel for the bacteria that live in the large intestine, encouraging them to proliferate. "The more fiber you eat, the more diversity you're going to have," Dr. Lee says.

One study compared the high-fiber diet of many South African men to the low-fiber diet typical of African American men. The study showed improvement in numerous inflammatory markers among the South Africans.

But the improvement comes with a drawback: "The more gas you'll have, too, unfortunately," Dr. Lee says.

That's right, fiber can cause flatulence. As with many other things in health, this one involves a trade-off.

12

HOW MANY GLASSES OF WINE CAN
I DRINK ON A FRIDAY NIGHT?

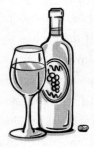

Let's start with the official suggestions. The Dietary Guidelines for Americans suggest limiting alcohol consumption to one drink a day for women and two per day for men. The Canadian guidelines are a little more lenient: no more than two drinks most days for women, for a total of ten drinks a week. Men are allowed fifteen drinks a week, with a limit of three drinks in one day.

My friends who are experts in this area say that's about right. For example, Dr. David Levy, an MD and the CEO of EHE, enjoys two glasses of wine with his dinner. He would let you get away with anywhere from two to four on a Friday night. His colleague, Dr. Tania Elliott, EHE's chief medical officer, is more conservative. "Night of the week doesn't matter," she says. "A glass of wine with dinner or a periodic cocktail is okay—all in moderation." What Dr. Elliott cautions against is saving up your consumption throughout the week and then "catching up" on Friday night with five drinks. "That's called binge drinking and can be just as much of a risk factor for alcoholism as drinking every day," she says.

Humans have had a conflicted relationship with alcohol for a long time. Archaeologists have discovered stone jugs thought to be intended to store fermented beverages dating back to Neolithic times, around 10,000 BC. One of the earliest popular drinks was fermented honey and water, which is known as mead. Residue from wine has been found in containers dating back to 5000 BC. Did the people who drank from those containers regret it the next morning? Or were they able to limit themselves to one or two drinks and feel good about consuming something with cancer-fighting antioxidants and, at least in moderation, properties associated with decreased risk of heart attack, stroke, and type 2 diabetes?

The idea that a little alcohol provides benefits dates back many years, too. For example, the nineteenth-century French chemist Louis Pasteur called wine "the most healthful and most hygienic of beverages." Pasteur's declaration made sense in his day, when water was often contaminated with harmful bacteria or parasites. But today the health benefits of moderate alcohol consumption are controversial. These days, if I were going to call something the most healthy of beverages, I'd likely go with water.

Every so often, the media gets excited about the latest epidemiological study that associates moderate alcohol consumption with a longer life span or some other healthy advantage, such as a decreased risk of heart disease. A glass of red wine a day is a suggested part of the Mediterranean diet, which has been shown to have all sorts of life-extending benefits. The theory is that alcohol may raise the levels of "good" cholesterol in the blood and that a small daily dose of alcohol lowers the blood's tendency to clot.

It's important to note, though, that these studies are correlative rather than causative. In other words, they don't actually prove that alcohol *causes* people to live longer, just that people with longer lives may enjoy a glass of wine each day. It's completely possible that some other, unrelated third factor accounts for the association. Perhaps the causative factor is the stress relief. There's something social and relaxing about savoring a bottle of wine with friends, and enjoying life may help prolong it. Personally, I like the idea that a bottle of wine is the perfect size for two people to share. Depending on the size of your pour, two people can get about two glasses each from a bottle—well within the guideline's single-night health recommendation.

As with so many things, balance is key. Even if it does have some benefits in moderation, alcohol is essentially a toxin. It's processed by the liver, and too much exposure to alcohol can harm the liver over time. Pregnant women should avoid consuming alcohol. There's some indication that a drink a day raises the risk of developing breast cancer in women and of atrial fibrillation in anyone who drinks moderately. Sure, having one drink a day can decrease blood pressure—but studies show that consuming more alcohol, such as three or four drinks a day, can elevate it.

There are two other concerns when it comes to alcohol consumption. First is the calorie question. Alcohol is a calorie-dense liquid; a shot of hard liquor has about 100 calories, a glass of wine 130, and a beer about 150. And alcohol portion sizes are increasing.

"Order a beer at a sporting event, and at some venues they'll give you a container that holds twenty ounces," says Dr. Steven Hirsch, one of Medcan's doctors. "You go to a restaurant now, they ask you whether you want a six- or a nine-ounce glass of wine—if you get the nine-ounce, that's almost two servings of wine."

Plus, an after-work drink can set up a cycle of indulgence in which it's not just the calories from the alcohol that can get problematic. People consume all sorts of foods with their alcohol. Cheese with wine. Salty snacks with a beer during a hockey or football game. All of that can add up quickly.

The other issue, of course, is with people who aren't able to control their drinking. That's a tough thing for some to confront. Plenty of high performers come to a point where one or two drinks a night is turning into many more. There's a work hard/play hard ethos in some job sectors that can be problematic.

Is alcohol affecting your job performance? Family relationships? Self-esteem? If that's the case, it may be time to change your relationship with alcohol. Professionals can help ease the transition from a life with alcohol to one without. Many people who abstain entirely find regular group meetings helpful. A web search for "Alcoholics Anonymous" will put one in touch with all sorts of people who live wonderful and full lives, completely sober.

To sum up, if you *do* drink in moderate amounts, continue with your judicious, limited intake, being careful not to exceed more than two or three glasses in a single night or binge on the weekends. If you don't drink at all, you shouldn't start drinking expressly for the health benefits, because the relationship of cost to benefit is close to even. "Don't drink alcohol as a way to get healthy," says Dr. Hirsch. "There are better ways to get healthy."

13

IS IT POSSIBLE TO EAT
WELL ON THE ROAD?

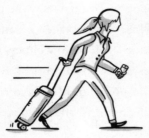

The short answer here is "yes, but it's difficult."

I spend a lot of time in airplanes and hotels, dashing from airport to airport, grabbing many of my meals in restaurants or at fast-food kiosks. If statistics are correct, plenty of people are like me, in terms of the frequency with which they're eating out. Research shows that men and women in industrialized nations are eating at restaurants and fast-food establishments more than ever. It used to be commonplace to prepare a lunch at home and take it to work; nowadays, rather than brown-bagging it, many of us grab our lunches at a coffee shop, a fast-food stand, or a lunch counter.

A 2012 USDA report showed that the proportion of calories Americans get from restaurants and fast-food outlets has almost doubled in recent decades, from 18 percent in 1977–78 to 32 percent by 2008. And I bet the trend has continued since then. That's a problem, because food in restaurants typically has higher levels of saturated fat, more sodium, and more calories than food prepared at home. In fact, for every meal eaten away from home, one's average caloric intake increases by 134 calories. Effectively, the more you eat out, the worse your diet tends to be.

So what to do?

When I'm away from home, I use a number of different rules to guide my eating. The rules are necessary because people can become more vulnerable to developing bad habits while they're on the road.

"When you're traveling, you're weaker, because you're outside of your normal circumstances," Medcan Wellness Clinic medical director Dr. Alain Sotto explains. "You don't have your friends, your coworkers, your family around you. Maybe you're a few time zones away, and your circadian rhythm's off, so you're not sleeping well. The body's willpower is reduced."

That means you're much more tempted to indulge when traveling: to have a few more glasses of wine, to have dessert, to grab the chips out of the hotel minibar. Which is why rules help.

Oddly, one of the best eat-well tips that I use when traveling has only a tangential relationship with food. It's this: exercise. Do it every day you're traveling. I'll often try to do it right after I check in to my hotel, because I've been breathing airplane and airport air for hours and nothing refreshes and refocuses me like getting outside and going for a run. Exercising is also a great mood booster. It can boost your willpower and help you sleep better. Exercise can help you make better decisions—about food, sure, but about everything else, too.

Now for actual eating. If there's fish or chicken as a menu option, that's what you should eat. Avoid eating the buns or rolls from the bread basket. The typical restaurant plate amounts to half starch—mashed potatoes, pasta, rice, or fries—with maybe a quarter of vegetable and a quarter of meat. But you can always ask the server to switch around the portions so that half of your plate is vegetables. And fries don't count as vegetables. In fact, avoid fries altogether. Make sure that each plate of food you eat has more green (vegetables) than red (meat).

In terms of drinks, a great way to start the day is with a protein shake, particularly if you're exercising. If you're thirsty during the day, try sparkling water because the carbonation will make you feel as though you're having something of substance, which, in turn, makes you less likely to snack on junk food. Plus the water helps with hydration. It's best to avoid alcohol on airplanes. The alcohol dehydrates, and if you abstain on the plane, you can save the glass of wine for when you're around others, giving it a social value.

One of Medcan's physician road warriors, Dr. Steven Hirsch, tries to eat a piece of fruit a half hour before any restaurant meal. "Doesn't matter what sort of fruit," he says. "Banana, apple, orange, a handful of blueberries. It dulls your appetite and enables you to think more clearly because you're not starving."

Another strategy is to avoid restaurants as much as possible when traveling. Try to get at least some of your meals in grocery stores. In the produce section, you can pick up some fruit, baby carrots, and snap peas, then head to the prepared food aisle for a packaged salad with chicken. The leftover carrots and snap peas go into the hotel minibar for snacks. Or if you want something more substantial to snack on, pack almonds, which are much healthier than the potato chips and pretzels that often come in the minibars.

Traveling in automobiles may be even trickier than by air when it comes to maintaining a healthy diet. Though the food found in rest stops does seems to be getting incrementally healthier, I would suggest some planning ahead when taking any lengthy road trip. Prepare some sandwiches. Cut up some vegetables. There's just too much likelihood of finding yourself hungry in a suburb or town where the only option is one fast-food drive-through or another.

Finally, if you're trying to adhere to some form of eating regimen—for example, if you're in training or you're hoping to lose some weight—and you slip up, don't beat yourself up. At Medcan, the doctor who runs our weight management clinic, Dr. David Macklin, often deals with people who go off their diets while traveling. The key, he says, is what happens next. Be resilient. Don't use the slip-up as an excuse to tank your entire eating regimen. Pick yourself up, dust yourself off, and return to your eating plan the next day. After all, eating well on the road is possible with these rules of thumb, but nobody's perfect.

14

DOES IT MATTER IF I EAT LOCAL?

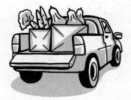

"Eating local" means trying to consume fruits, vegetables, and other whole foods that have been grown near where you live. There are various definitions of what constitutes local. One extreme is food grown yourself. Another is food produced within a hundred miles of your home. Other definitions are satisfied so long as the food comes from a place within your state or province—or even the same side of your country.

There are two main reasons to eat local: one, the approach can benefit the planet; two, it can also be good for your health.

Let's discuss the environmental reason first. Different foods extract very different environmental costs from the earth. Producing food for Earth's human population accounts for a quarter of all greenhouse gas emissions, according to a 2016 study out of Oxford University's Martin Programme on the Future of Food.

My nutrition staff uses the following rule: the higher you eat on the food chain, the higher the environmental cost. An ear of corn or a sprig of wheat is lower on the food chain than the chick or calf that eats it—and costs the earth less to produce, as well.

Increasing the number of plants you eat is not the same as eating local. But eating more green than red, as I think of it, is an important way to start considering the environmental costs of one's diet.

Once you start thinking about the sustainability of your food, you're apt to confront some troubling facts about its origin. Such as your grocery store's position as the final link in a global logistics chain. Those pears in your produce basket may come from South Africa. Mangoes and avocados may have been raised in Mexican soil. California produces 99 percent of US-grown almonds, which require enormous amounts of water—about a gallon per almond—and account for about a tenth of California's agricultural water use. Similarly, a pound of Chilean-grown avocados can consume 96.8 gallons of water, while the average water consumption elsewhere to grow a pound of avocados is 28.4 gallons.

One way to get a better sense of the origins of fruits and vegetables is by shopping at farmer's markets, an experience that can provide an education in the seasonality of food. Tomatoes, corn, and strawberries are seasonal harvests in most of the United States and Canada. Shopping at a farmer's market that features locally grown and produced foods is a reminder of what's in season and what isn't.

Which brings us to the second reason to eat local: the health implications. Consuming the bounty of nearby farms can improve the diversity of one's diet, which is healthy. "Seasonality produces variety," says Dr. Michael Parkinson, the former president of the American College of Preventive Medicine who is an enthusiastic consumer of locally produced fruits and vegetables. "Certain foods grow at certain times of the year—and those changing crops create variety in available micronutrients in a complimentary way."

Seasonality can also present its share of problems. During winter in Canada and much of the United States, it can be difficult to get the full range of vitamins and nutrients from strictly local foods. The only places where citrus fruits such as oranges and grapefruit are local are Florida and California. Those of us who live in the north can get our vitamin C from cabbage or cauliflower in the fall and strawberries in the summer—or we can relax a bit and eat some Florida grapefruit or California oranges.

Though eating local is important, it's important to acknowledge the benefits of a global economy. Try to continue shopping for foods that are in season during the colder months—potatoes, squash, parsnips, and cabbage, for instance—but don't feel too guilty when you eat mandarin oranges in December.

What I'd suggest is that you eat local when it's possible. Local farmer's markets can provide an education in food. They can also be a lot of fun. Their produce costs a little more than what's at the nearest big-box food retailer, but you're also supporting local growers and benefiting the environment. Try to eat local when you can, but don't worry too much if you break the rule when the inconvenience outweighs the nutritional benefits.

15

HOW CAN I PRACTICE MINDFUL EATING?

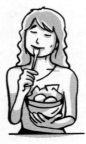

So often, when thinking about healthful eating, we focus on the "what" of our diet—the precise mix of fats, carbs, and proteins that we ingest during the course of a day. What many of us fail to consider are the circumstances around our eating; that is, the "when" and the "how." But the timing of our meals and how we eat them may be just as important as what we put into our mouths.

Thinking about *how* you eat as much as *what* you eat is an approach that many in the nutrition field call "mindful eating." It's based on the tenets of mindfulness, a form of meditation that places the emphasis on experiencing life as it happens to us. Some people call it "being in the moment."

The way many urban professionals eat is pretty much the opposite of mindfulness. Breakfast might be ordered in a drive-through lane. The coffee is gulped, the egg-and-muffin sandwich swallowed fast. Or maybe it's a bagel on the way to the subway. Or maybe you skip eating breakfast altogether. Lunch is often at one's desk, swallowed between emails. I'm as guilty of this as anyone—many of the calories I ingest are from smoothies that I consume on the go.

Mindful eating encourages one to slow down, experience, and enjoy the act of eating, paying attention not only to the food eaten but also to the circumstances around it: the hunger signals that prompted the act of eating in the first place, the taste and texture of the food, the body's response to swallowing the food, the satiety sensation that, ideally, prompts the conclusion of the meal.

The idea, then, particularly for problematic eaters, is to find out *why* you're eating the way you do, with a view to changing any bad habits. The approach can provide remarkable benefits to people who are struggling with their weight—sometimes ironing out a few triggers is all that's required to drop some pounds.

Take the help provided by Medcan dietitian Stefania Palmeri. She walked a client through his daily eating habits, and the encounter went something like this.

"So what do you eat for breakfast?" she said.

"Usually nothing," he said. "I don't have time. Instead, I get up, I maybe grab a coffee, and then it's off to work."

"What's the first thing you *do* eat?" asked Palmeri.

The gentleman told Palmeri about his habit of grabbing a cinnamon bun in the cafeteria on his way to a daily 11 a.m. meeting.

Next, Palmeri and the client discussed lunch—which tended to overcompensate for his missed morning meal. He ate a huge lunch from one of the fast-food restaurants in a strip mall near his building. Poutine, burgers, Greek food, noodle bowls—what it was varied depending on the food court's daily special, but one thing was certain: he ate a lot of it.

See the problem? Starving the body of food in the morning drops blood sugar levels and increases cortisol levels, which prompts the body to start breaking down muscle mass for energy. Then eating a big meal at lunch creates something called a "hyperinsulemic response"—a spike in insulin levels that prevents the satiety hormone, ghrelin, from shutting off the appetite, leading you to eat more than you otherwise might.

That brings us to a key principle of healthful eating behaviors: no one makes good food choices when they're hungry. If you ignore the body's signals about when to eat and stop eating, when you *do* eat, you'll be famished and consume too much.

Mindful eating is about more than just eating timing and avoiding becoming too hungry, however. Another key habit is to avoid looking at food as a reward—to realize that what we're craving, as one mindful eating workbook says, is "the feeling that results from eating, not the food itself."

By slowing down and paying attention to the circumstances that surround eating, as well as the act of eating itself, the techniques of mindful eating can help you get into touch with your relationship with food; to realize when one is hungry, as well as when one is satisfied. As the director of Medcan's weight management program, Dr. David Macklin, points out, people who eat when they're hungry and stop when they're satisfied are more likely to lose weight and keep it off. They're also less likely to become overweight in the first place.

The ultimate goal? To enjoy food without obsessing over it.

So consider the following techniques, each of which are drawn from mindful eating practices:

- When you notice feelings of hunger coming on, eat a nutritious snack.
- Stop eating when you're two-thirds full, because it takes twenty minutes for the brain to register the satiety sent from your gut.

- Eat slowly, and chew each bite of food well.
- Eat with others, because it makes the meal more enjoyable and you tend to eat more slowly.
- Try not to do anything else while you're eating.

Mindful eating will not fix every aspect of a poor diet. Someone who exists on a diet of cheese and ice cream will eventually have to make changes to the *kind* of food he or she eats. But it's never a bad thing to pay attention to the circumstances in which you consume your food and that may play a factor in your overeating. Enjoy and savor each bite of food you take.

16

IS IT POSSIBLE TO CONSUME TOO *LITTLE* SODIUM?

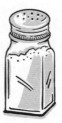

The big worry about sodium is consuming too much of the stuff. Approximately 25 percent of North Americans have high blood pressure, a key risk factor for cardiovascular disease. Consuming too much sodium can elevate blood pressure, increasing the risk of a heart attack or stroke. What's comparatively lesser known is that consuming too *little* sodium can be a problem as well. In fact, consuming too little sodium can also elevate the risk of a cardiovascular event.

Sodium and humanity go way back. We probably didn't eat much of the stuff back in Paleolithic times, when we were hunters and foragers. It was the advent of agriculture that brought salt into our diets. We first used salt to preserve perishable food during winter. Salt was so important to ancient humans that the Roman Empire provided its soldiers with money to purchase it.

Nowadays, when we think of salt and sodium, we think of the white crystals in the shaker that we sprinkle over our meals (table salt, a compound of the minerals sodium and chloride, is about 40 percent sodium; one teaspoon contains roughly 2,300 milligrams of sodium). But recent research suggests that only 5 percent of sodium consumption comes from salt added during a meal. Approximately 70 percent of it is consumed in prepared dishes, such as highly processed foods or in meals we consume at restaurants or fast-food outlets.

Lower sodium consumption is associated with lower blood pressure. Each additional gram of sodium you consume per day over and above 5 grams increases your systolic blood pressure by 2.63 mm Hg. (Systolic blood pressure is the first number mentioned in a measure such as 120 over 80 and reflects the pressure in the blood vessels as the heart beats.) That can be even greater for people who are considered "salt sensitive" because they have blood pressure that increases more than normal with salt intake.

Many medical professionals counsel their patients to limit their sodium intake. It makes sense. Cardiovascular disease remains the world's biggest killer, accounting for about a third of all deaths globally. And if decreasing sodium consumption can lower blood pressure, which in turn lowers the risk of cardiovascular disease, why not try to radically decrease how much salt you take in?

But there's a catch. Decreasing sodium consumption does work to decrease the risk of cardiovascular disease. But only to a point. One complicating factor is that the body requires a certain level of salt. Sodium is important to regulating the water content in cells and assists with the functioning of our nerves and muscles. Too little sodium intake activates a pathway called the renin-angiotensin-aldosterone system, which in turn may interfere with the regulation of fats in the blood. The end effect? Very low sodium intake can actually increase the risk of cardiovascular disease.

Once again, balance is key. Your cardiovascular disease risk increases if you ingest more than 6 grams of sodium per day, and it also increases if you consume less than 3 grams of sodium per day. The ideal lies in the middle, between 3 and 5 grams of sodium per day. Those who suffer from hypertension should aim for the lower end of the sweet spot, closer to 3 grams of sodium per day.

K-RATION

The mineral potassium helps the kidneys regulate fluid levels in the body in a way that helps control blood pressure—to such an extent that consuming potassium may counteract the effects of sodium. Foods that are high in potassium include winter squash, sweet potatoes, broccoli, and bananas.

There is still debate on this topic. The National Academy of Medicine, which sets guidelines for both the United States and Canada, specifies an upper limit for sodium intake of 2,300 milligrams per day for the general population. The American Heart Association suggests "an ideal limit" of 1,500 milligrams per day for most adults. And Hypertension Canada, which provides guidelines to doctors on how best to decrease patient blood pressure, once suggested a sodium target of 1,500 milligrams per day but elevated the target in 2013 because it was thought to be unrealistic for most people. Today the organization suggests that people who have high blood pressure "consider reducing sodium intake toward 2,000 mg per day."

It can be difficult to stay within the limits. For example, the breakfast sandwiches from your favorite coffee shop can contain more than 1,000 milligrams of sodium. A typical bag of plain potato chips has 170 milligrams of sodium per single-ounce serving, so an 8-ounce package has 1,360 milligrams. And a medium-sized order of fries from a fast-food restaurant contains 260 milligrams—before you sprinkle salt on it.

"Many people need to cut down their sodium intake, whether they have high blood pressure or not," says Leslie Beck, Medcan's director of food and nutrition. "The problem is our steady fare of highly processed foods and salt-laden restaurant meals. But focusing only on a single nutrient like sodium risks missing the forest for the trees. Instead, we should focus on eating fewer ultraprocessed foods and far more wholesome nutritious foods like vegetables, fruit, and whole grains."

I agree. If you do have high blood pressure, talk to your doctor and dietitian about a sodium level that's appropriate for you. Remember that the processed foods with the highest sodium content are things such as breads, salted meats, canned goods, snack foods, and fast foods. Watch how many breakfast sandwiches you eat on your way to work, and go easy on the soy sauce when you're out for sushi. A taste for salt is a learned behavior, and a moratorium on the flavoring can reset your taste buds so that you no longer crave it. In addition, consider flavoring what you eat with other things, such as lemon juice, herbs, and spices.

Even if you don't have high blood pressure, consider reducing the amount of heavily processed and restaurant food you eat, cooking at home more, and increasing the amount of plants in your diet—all of which are likely to reduce your sodium consumption, as well as help you eat better in general.

17

WHY ARE SO MANY FOOD
EXPERTS NUTS ABOUT NUTS?

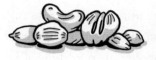

I keep a bowl of nuts on my kitchen counter. Throughout the course of a day, when I'm home, I'll take a little scoop of whatever happens to be in it—almonds, pecans, cashews, pistachios, maybe walnuts. The snack takes the edge off my hunger. But more than that, nuts have been proven to have numerous benefits for our health.

Nuts have undergone a remarkable resurgence in recent years. Years ago, people considered them a fatty snack, just a rung or two up the food ladder from junk food such as potato chips or nachos. Today they've been rehabilitated into a health food.

Several years ago, Harvard researchers analyzed data from two large, long-duration cohort studies on health professionals that followed the lifestyle choices of a combined 119,000 people over two decades. One thing they tracked was nut consumption. The Harvard researchers took the group of people, categorized them by the frequency with which they ate nuts, and then figured out how long those in each category lived—and if they had died, what had killed them.

The researchers found that nut consumption was associated with substantially lower rates of death. It didn't matter what sorts of nuts were consumed, whether a handful of peanuts (which are actually legumes, like peas) or tree nuts, such as almonds, cashews, walnuts, or pecans. The more nuts people ate—up to a single 1-ounce serving per day—the less heart disease they experienced, the less likely they were to contract cancer, and the less likely they were to suffer from major respiratory diseases.

Later studies have shown that nut consumption is associated with benefits for health conditions as varied as type 2 diabetes, metabolic syndrome, colon cancer, and high blood pressure. The Harvard Study doesn't prove causality; that is, the studies didn't prove that nut consumption prevented such health conditions. But the results are intriguing for the remarkable span of the benefits with which nuts are associated, including reduced levels of "bad" LDL cholesterol, better blood sugar regulation, and improved arterial function.

Nuts are a nutrient-dense food, which means that they cram lots of good things into a comparatively small package. They have a lot of fiber and plant protein, as well as such antioxidants as vitamin E, which is good for brain health, and folate, a B vitamin. They're also high in such minerals as potassium and magnesium. And they're full of other health-benefiting substances such as phytosterols, which help lower cholesterol and reduce inflammation.

"Nuts also contain an amino acid called L-arginine which can help make your arteries more flexible and prevent cholesterol plaque buildup," says EHE chief medical officer Dr. Tania Elliott.

The big criticism of nuts years ago was that they were chock full

NUTTIN' TO IT

A single serving of nuts is 1 ounce, or 28 grams. That amounts to the following quantities:

24 shelled almonds

8 medium Brazil nuts

18 cashews

20 hazelnuts or filberts

12 macadamia nuts

28 peanuts

20 pecan halves

40 pistachios

14 English walnut halves

of fat. But the fats that nuts contain are mostly the heart-healthy, unsaturated kind. In the Harvard study, higher nut consumption was associated with lower body mass index, and other studies have found that eating nuts was associated with reduced waist circumference and a decreased risk of obesity.

There isn't one "best" nut. Medcan registered dietitian Stefania Palmeri encourages her clients to mix up the sort of nuts they eat.

"Each nut carries a different benefit," she says. "Almonds are good for calcium. Brazil nuts have selenium in them. And walnuts have omega-3 fats."

That said, I would caution people to watch that they don't eat too many nuts. A cup of almonds has more than 800 calories, and other nuts are just as calorie dense. Medcan's Dr. Steven Hirsch suggests that his patients limit their consumption of nuts to "a handful" per day. Also, watch how the nuts are served. Control your intake of salted, candied, or sugared nuts. Leslie Beck, Medcan's director of food and nutrition, points out that roasting nuts can enhance their flavor without compromising their nutrient content.

And, most important, remember that all things are better in moderation. One member of my nutrition team, Alexandra Friel, was working with a client who wanted to lose 20 pounds. He'd dropped 15 already, but he just couldn't manage the final 5—until Alex went through the whole of his food consumption with him. It turned out that he was eating a cup and a half of nuts a day. In almonds, that added up to more than 1,200 calories. The final pounds became manageable once he scaled back his consumption to a single serving each day. Sometimes even nuts can be too much of a good thing!

Part Two

MOVE

I'VE NEVER EXERCISED REGULARLY BEFORE. WHERE DO I START?

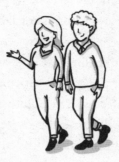

You probably have some vague sense that exercise is a good thing to do. But you may not realize just how good it is. Exercise is the single most effective lever to a long, healthy, and active life. It's important *now*. And it becomes even more important as you age.

Regular bouts of physical activity provide us with tangible benefits. Exercise decreases the risk of stroke as well as type 2 diabetes and colon and breast cancers. It lowers blood pressure and improves blood chemistry. It enhances insulin sensitivity and helps manage weight. And for older adults, exercise helps to maintain bone and muscle strength and reduces the risk of falling.

Then there are the unexpected benefits of exercise. Regularly engaging in physical activity can help counteract depression and anxiety. We sleep better when we exercise. It improves our sex lives and, particularly in men, our sexual function. It enhances our feelings of well-being and overall enjoyment of life. And a growing body of scientific evidence suggests that exercise also helps the brain, boosting cognitive function long into old age and pushing back such aging symptoms as dementia or other cognitive declines.

We're now realizing that exercise amounts to powerful medicine for the human body. In fact, there's a doctor in New York, an orthopedic surgeon named Dr. Jordan Metzl, who's become well known for hosting regular free workout sessions in public parks. A veteran of thirty marathons and eleven Ironman triathlons at last count, as well as the author of several books, he's a self-described "exercise warrior" who has made it his life's mission to encourage his fellow doctors to "prescribe" exercise to their patients.

"There is no more effective, safe, and basically risk-free drug," he says of exercise. "It works for every single person, rich or poor, young or old. There's no other drug like it. [Exercise] is, in fact, the most potent, safe, effective medicine across the spectrum of the human condition, and we need to make sure everybody takes this drug every day of their lives."

But how to start? The first thing is to pick something you'll be likely to do.

"If you're someone who hates to swim," says Dr. I-Min Lee, an MD and epidemiologist, "and you say, 'I'm going to swim to get my exercise'—that's never going to stick. You have to find out what it is that you like so you can do it and not feel like it's a chore."

Whatever activity you choose, make sure it's something that can become a habit.

"Most of us don't get up in the morning and think 'Should I brush my teeth or should I not?' You just do it—it's become a habit," says Dr. Lee. "Exercise should be the same thing."

Be careful not to start out too hard. That elevates the risk of injury, and an early injury can turn you off exercising for years.

"A lot of people who have never before worked out think of exercise as something that's difficult to do," says Geralyn Coopersmith, an exercise physiologist who worked as Nike's global director of performance and fitness training. "They think it requires equipment. Special shoes. Workout clothes. But that's not the case at all. When you're starting out exercising, you want to choose something that provides the minimal barrier to entry. The form of exercise that most fits into your life and doesn't require a lot of equipment."

So what might your first forays into exercise look like?

How about walking?

That's right. The same thing you use to get from the car to the mall. That gets you from your couch to the washroom. Walking is the world's most universal exercise. Pretty much everyone knows how to do it. It's free, and you can do it anywhere in the world.

EXERCISE, THE NATURAL REMEDY

Exercise provides us with the physical activity that we evolved to do every day, just to survive. Previous generations had physical activity built into their daily lives. They didn't *need* a gym. Now we've engineered all of the physical activity out of our day-to-day existence. With our tablet computers, same-day delivery services, Roomba motorized vacuum cleaners, and supersized drinks, we're becoming uncomfortably close to the human beings satirized at the end of the Pixar movie *WALL-E*, who glide about in hovering chairs, their every need met, screens inches from their faces, sipping vat-sized sugary drinks as they go.

Our bodies evolved to need the physical activity that was a part of previous generations' everyday lives. Even though our day-to-day lives have changed, we still need that physical activity to stay healthy. We're designed for a certain amount of activity, and if we don't get it, things start to go awry. All this talk of exercise is just figuring out how to put back into our lives all the activity we used to get naturally.

I take pains to incorporate walking into my workday. Rather than staying cooped up in an office for a meeting with a colleague, I'll often suggest we head outside and walk around the neighborhood. I'll also head out on a walk during phone meetings.

"Get up and walk out one direction for fifteen minutes," Coopersmith suggests, "then turn around and come back."

That's a half-hour walk. That's an achievement. The nice thing about a half-hour walk is that it's relatively easy to schedule, particularly if you use that time to connect with friends by phone or in person.

If you're just starting out, set a goal to go for five half-hour walks within some achievable period—try two weeks to start. Once you've accomplished the five walks, assess how they've gone. Do you feel worse than when you started? I doubt it. In fact, I bet you feel better because you've accomplished something. Not only that, but five walks are all it takes to start providing you with fitness benefits.

So what's next? One possibility is incorporating intervals into the walking—boost your pace to a brisk walk for a block or two, then ease off. Keep doing that until you've incorporated six to ten intervals throughout the course of the walk. Once you're able to get through the half-hour walk, with intervals and without breathing heavily, try working in some strength-building exercises. (We'll get to precisely what strength-building exercises you should try later on in this part.)

And if you weren't able to meet that goal of five walks in two weeks, I love the suggestion of Dr. Robert Ross, an exercise physiologist at Queen's University. "Get a dog," he says. His logic? Even if walking isn't something you're particularly inclined to do, owning a dog gets you outside and moving no matter what—because several times a day, you need to get moving.

CAN STAYING ACTIVE STAVE OFF AGING?

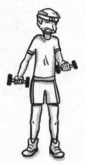

Aging sucks, or, at least, certain *aspects* of aging suck. For example, the progress of time alone is thought to diminish the mass of your muscles by 3 to 5 percent with each decade that passes after the age of 30.

The process of age-related diminishing muscle mass is known as sarcopenia, and the conventional wisdom suggests that it happens because of aging. But recently people in the exercise sciences have begun to wonder whether sarcopenia may be caused by something else: inactivity. The implication is that if we stay active, we just may be able to ward off the reduced mobility and strength we associate with aging.

For example, in one University of Pittsburgh study, researchers analyzed cross-section magnetic resonance imaging (MRI) of thighs belonging to three groups: masters triathletes in their seventies, normal senior citizens, and younger athletes in their forties.

The athletes in their forties had thighs that were bursting with muscle. Thighs belonging to regular 70-year-old senior citizens looked a lot different—they were mostly fatty tissue wrapped around an insubstantial core of atrophied muscle. And the 70-year-old triathletes? Their thighs looked the same as those belonging to the 40-year-old athletes.

So how can you stave off the aging process? The answer is exercise; simple physical activity and movement. Dr. James Aw, Medcan's chief medical officer, says that we should be thinking of the decision to exercise today in terms similar to investing for retirement. "The trouble is, many of the people obsessively tracking the worth of their stock portfolios and RRSP balances pay little attention to *health*. They don't exercise because they're too busy working toward their retirements. Which makes no sense. If these folks *really* thought ahead, they'd understand that exercise is just as important to a healthy retirement as saving up money."

Dr. Mark Tarnopolsky of McMaster University is a world expert in the ways that exercise fights aging. He also endorses that kind of thinking. "How does everyone want to die?" he asks. "I think you want to be independent, with your spouse. You want to go to bed at night, have your last lovemaking session, and not wake up in the morning. You go from being functional to dead. The last thing I think people want is a slow decline where you become debilitated."

Exercise, he says, is how you go about avoiding that slow decline. In fact, his studies have shown that it really is possible to stave off the aging process—and possibly even to reverse it.

One of Tarnopolsky's major research topics is mitochondria, the powerhouses of cells. For most of our lives, mitochondria convert fuel, such as glucose and fat, into energy. Mitochondria are a bit finicky, however. Like the engine of a high-performing sports car, they can break down. At first when that happens, the cell repairs them. But as we get older, our cells start losing the ability to make those repairs, and the mitochondria stay broken.

Tarnopolsky and his colleagues subscribe to something called "the mitochondrial theory of aging," which says that many of the problems we associate with getting older—such as weaker muscles, more brittle bones, receding hairlines, wrinkles, and gray hair— might happen because the mitochondria go unrepaired. And according to Tarnopolsky, the best way to ensure that our mitochondria stay healthy is by exercising.

The best news is that it's never too late to start. "Even if you start exercising in your fifties, your sixties, or your seventies," Dr. I-Min Lee says, "you still gain longevity relative to people in your age group." Start younger, and you gain more years, she points out. I love the way she puts it: "You're not just adding years to your life— you're adding life to your years."

So the most effective lever to achieving that healthy last ten years is through maintaining your fitness today. How do you want the last ten years of your life to look? Each of us has a choice: head toward a future of hospitals, wheelchairs, and doctor visits; or start exercising, and be able to keep up with our grandkids. Because the final act of your life should also be the best one.

3

WHAT'S A BASIC STRENGTH-BUILDING RESISTANCE WORKOUT THAT ANYONE CAN DO PRETTY MUCH ANYWHERE?

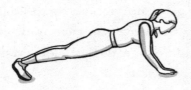

The problem with resistance training is that many people think it's difficult. They associate it with weights and complex equipment. But you don't need fancy machines to perform an exercise circuit that will build strength and give you a decent workout. That's because you can use your body itself as the weight you lift.

Here is a range of strength-building exercises that you can do anywhere from a hotel room to a cottage to a conference room. Together they're designed to provide a full-body workout that will increase the likelihood that you'll stay active and injury free long into your senior years.

PUSH-UP

Maybe the best known and most popular of the body-weight exercises, push-ups are great because they build muscle from the pectorals to the deltoids and on into the triceps. Plus they're essentially a plank, so they're working your abdominal muscles, too.

The standard version involves lying on your belly with your hands palm down on either side of the shoulders—your elbows should form about a ninety-degree angle. Start by pushing your torso, held straight from shoulders to toes, into the air until your arms are straight. Then slowly lower your torso back to the ground. Lead the descent with your chest, rather than your head or pelvis.

Don't get discouraged if you can't do a standard push-up at first. Easier variations are also fun to do, and push-ups are one of those exercises where rapid improvement is possible.

PROGRESSION: If it's your first time doing push-ups regularly, start by leaning on a wall and pushing out from that. Once you're able to perform 10 standing push-ups like that, move on to placing your hands on something that sees your body closer to the horizontal—a heavy dining room table or the edge of a sofa or a coffee table. Using stairs is also a good option. Once you can easily do 10 push-ups at that level, move on to the standard push-up on the ground. And if you're looking to make the exercise even more difficult, you can move on to decline push-ups, where your toes are elevated above your hands, with the resistance increasing the higher the toes' elevation.

REPS: Each workout, aim for three sets of 10 push-ups each.

STEP-UP

This exercise is easy to do anywhere—all you need is a difference in elevation, namely, a step. It works numerous different muscle groups in the legs, from the quadriceps to the buttocks' gluteus maximus. The step-up is preferable to the squat because the motion of the step-up develops balance in addition to leg strength.

To perform it, stand before a step and place your right foot on it. Then step up to the higher elevation until your left foot is next to your right. Lower your left foot to the ground where it started. Repeat that ten times and then switch legs.

The front leg should be doing the majority of the work, so avoid pushing off the back leg. Leaning your body over your front leg will isolate the glutes and may be a better technique for someone with knee issues. If your front foot doesn't have the room to stand fully on the higher step, you can always stand sideways.

PROGRESSION: There are a few ways to make step-ups more difficult. You can elevate the height of the step until your knee is ninety degrees at the exercise's start. Don't go any higher than that, though, or you risk injury. If you want a greater challenge, try adding weight to your body. If you don't have dumbbells, consider using a backpack filled with books or a laptop computer, or simply hold evenly weighted shopping bags, one in each hand.

REPS: Aim for 10 step-ups with one leg, then switch legs and perform another set of 10, for a total of three sets on either side. If you notice that one side is weaker, always begin with that side.

ONE-ARMED ROW

Every strength-building circuit should include a pulling motion to work back muscles such as the latissimus dorsi and rhomboids. Exercising the back balances the forces on the shoulder and helps avoid developing a strength imbalance.

To perform the exercise, find a flat surface that is about the height of your knee. A stable coffee table, bench, or couch works well. Begin by placing a weight—ideally a dumbbell—on the ground beside you. If you don't have a dumbbell available, any heavy object will work; for example, if you're in a hotel room, you could use the bed as the support and a bottle of minibar wine as the weight.

Set your right knee on the surface. Place the palm of your right hand flat on the same surface so that your back is bent over and parallel to the ground; your left foot should remain flat on the ground. Dangle your left arm so it's at a right angle to your back, then pull the weight up toward your ribs until it's even with the torso. Ensure that the shoulder blade pulls back as the hand comes up and that it moves forward as the hand descends. Repeat that ten times and then switch sides.

PROGRESSION: The difficulty of this exercise increases with the amount of weight you lift. If you don't have a dumbbell available, start off holding a can of pop, a book, or a carton of milk, and once you're able to perform 10 reps comfortably, increase the weight. You can also purchase rubber exercise tubing at any fitness store. Step on one end and pull up with your arm on the other to simulate a free weight.

REPS: Aim for three sets of 10 with each arm.

HIP RAISE

Also known as the butt lift or bridge, the idea behind the hip raise is to target the gluteus muscles of your buttocks and your lower back muscles. It also strengthens the hamstrings. It's a bit of an unconventional motion, but it's important because it mitigates some of the damage done to the body by sitting in a desk chair all day.

Start by lying down on the floor, back down. Raise your knees so your feet are flat on the floor, about a foot apart from each other. Thrust your hips into the air until your body is an even plank running from your shoulders to your knees. Hold for a few seconds, then lower your hips slowly to the ground.

PROGRESSION: Once you're able to perform 10 repetitions comfortably, increase the difficulty by holding the hips in the bridge position and bringing one knee toward your chest—a motion known as the marching glute bridge. Set the one leg down, then bring the other knee to the chest. Once you're able to perform 10 reps of that motion, try single-leg hip bridges.

REPS: Do three sets of 10. If you're doing single-leg hip bridges, do 10 for each leg.

SIDE PLANK

Many exercise circuits include the standard plank to work the abdominal muscles. But you're already working that muscle group with the push-ups. So why not try side planks, which isolate the parts of the core that we don't often target—the obliques, hip abductors, abs, and glutes. The idea is to stabilize the hip, pelvis, and spine by strengthening the muscles around them, which will in turn protect your back from excessive loads.

If it's your first time doing the exercise, lie on one side with your knees bent at ninety degrees. With your forearm perpendicular to your body, raise your torso up on one elbow. Try to keep as straight a line as possible from the knees through to the head. Hold the pose for at least 10 seconds, then lower yourself to the ground.

• • •

PROGRESSION: After holding the pose for 10 seconds at a time, take a break and repeat. Over time, increase the time you hold the pose. Once you're able to hold the pose for 90 seconds, increase the difficulty by moving the lower support from your knees to your feet. Your top leg should be set forward about a foot's length from the rear foot. Once you're able to manage that for 90 seconds, increase the difficulty by repeatedly tapping your top leg ahead and behind your lower foot.

REPS: Try to conduct five reps of the 10-second hold on each side of the body, whether you're supporting yourself on your knees or your feet. Once you incorporate toe taps, try to perform a total of 20 taps before you switch to the opposite side of the body.

Practice each of these exercises on its own; then, once you have a good sense of the movements required, perform the exercises as a circuit. Start with a set of push-ups, followed by a set of step-ups for each leg, one-armed rows on each arm, and hip raises. Go through the circuit until you've performed three sets of each exercise. Finally, do the side planks.

Congratulations—you've just completed a whole-body resistance-training exercise circuit session that will help keep your body strong and your back straight and injury free for years to come!

IS EXERCISE A MEDICINE?

Consider the story of Carl Spiess, 52, who started developing health problems in his early forties. One of the big issues he had was acid reflux, a burning sensation in the diaphragm caused by stomach acid climbing up into the esophagus. Spiess went to see his family doctor, who sent him to a specialist who suggested surgery. The specialist wanted to slice off a length of Spiess's abdominal muscle and wrap it around his upper esophagus, so that it could prevent the stomach acid from rising up into his throat.

Then there was his back, which Spiess had hurt trying to lift a stuck snowmobile. There were days his back hurt so much it was difficult to get out of bed. Late in the day, his employees would come into his office and find him lying on the floor, face to the ceiling, because that was the only position that didn't hurt. Guess what a specialist suggested to solve that problem? That's right: surgery.

Spiess figured he should exhaust all possibilities before he went under the knife. He went to get a second opinion, and this doctor had told him that he might see some benefits from starting an exercise regimen. So Spiess started working out, performing resistance exercises to build his muscle strength.

As he kept up with his fitness regimen, a remarkable thing happened; the acid reflux disappeared entirely. One day, one of his employees walked into his office and said, "We haven't seen you on the ground recently, Carl—has your back improved?" Not only had it improved, but the back pain had disappeared. That year was the first one in which Spiess didn't have to take a single sick day.

Years later, Spiess has kept up his workouts. He's maintained an active lifestyle; in fact, he's taken up windsurfing and runs a popular blog chronicling his new sports adventures. His story illustrates the power of exercise as a prescription. The working out helped his core strength, which eased his back pain. It also decreased his stress—and the decreased stress levels took care of the acid reflux. What happens when you actually do take exercise as a medicine? Your life improves.

4

I CAN BARELY FIND TIME TO DO MY LAUNDRY. HOW CAN I INCORPORATE EXERCISE INTO MY LIFE?

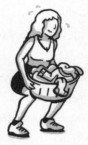

Everyone struggles to find the time to exercise. I get it: we're all busy. I have a friend, Bill Stauffer, who has run a number of well-known fitness brands, such as Equinox, SoulCycle, and now Flywheel Sports, a New York–based fitness company that operates spinning and barre boutiques. But even Bill has to take special steps to ensure that he fits his workouts into his schedule.

Bill has a routine he goes through each week. When he wakes up on Sunday morning, the first thing he does is reach for his computer and create fitness appointments for himself through the next seven days. He moves the little colored squares around on his calendar app until he has five separate blocks of exercise time per week. "Tons of stuff might pop up in the course of the week—but I hold that time," he says.

Let's say you've set a goal to exercise three times a week for the next three months. The first thing to do is to make it difficult to get out of those exercise sessions. One trick that many successful longtime exercisers use is to work out first thing in the morning, when your reserves of willpower are high and before there's anything else going on at work or at home. The night before, pack your gym bag, pick out your workout clothes and leave them in a convenient place, and as soon as your alarm sounds, spring up and go for your workout. You could hit the gym, attend an early class, or just get out for an early bike ride or jog.

The *when* becomes a lot easier if you've chosen some good exercise partners. A fitness goal becomes a lot more achievable if you do it with someone else. So think about setting up an appointment with a friend to attend a certain fitness session. "I'll meet you for the noon boot camp class on Monday, Wednesday, and Friday," you might say—and now you have an incentive to show up. After all, you don't want to disappoint your friend.

Nor does it have to be a friend. Say your job has moved you to a new city where you don't know any potential exercise partners. In that case, consider making an appointment with a fitness trainer, kind of as a surrogate friend. Or you could join a free local running club. Or a sports league. Most urban centers have options for everything from soccer to hockey, flag football, and ultimate Frisbee. The fact that your teammates are counting on you to show up creates the motivation to get you there.

So make a commitment to someone else—that's number one. Another important principle is to make exercise fun.

"I've been in the industry for well over thirty years," says Paul Juris, chief science officer at the sports equipment manufacturer Cybex International. "I've seen everything come and go. If you think about the types of activities and fitness that have stood the test of time, what's common to all of them is that they are *group* activities.

They're not just exercise. They're a group of people doing something *together*."

The general idea, then, is to choose forms of fitness that you enjoy. A lot of challenges exist for exercise in a world of Netflix, movies, and drive-through everything. The first step is to recognize that exercise is an important and necessary part of your health. If you've done that, take the time to create a strategy for working exercise into your life. Schedule your workouts, connect with a fitness community, and create incentives that will make you commit to them. If you do that, you'll look forward to your workouts, and you'll figure out reasons to make them happen.

5

HOW MANY DAYS A WEEK
SHOULD I WORK OUT?

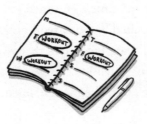

Ask experts how much exercise a person should do in a week, and they'll likely quote the American College of Sports Medicine's official, ideal guideline: thirty minutes of moderate exercise a day for at least five days a week. It can be half that if you're dialing the intensity up to a vigorous exercise. The ACSM also recommends resistance training—basically, exercises that build strength (what we used to call weight training)—two or three times a week.

That regimen could easily entail five and a half hours of exercise a week. But meeting the guidelines doesn't actually require that much time. In fact, if your schedule is full yet you're intent on adhering to the guidelines, it's possible to fulfill the spirit of the guidelines in just one hour and fifteen minutes over seven days.

The secret is circuit training, which turns your resistance training into vigorous cardio exercise by keeping your heart rate elevated. In other words, you can create a workout with strength-building exercises that improves your endurance at the same time.

One way to do that is by cutting out the breaks between

resistance sets and alternating among exercises that work different major muscle groups. For example, maybe you start a twenty-five-minute circuit with squats, which work the muscles in your thighs and buttocks, among many others. Then you move on to push-ups to exercise your chest, shoulder, and arm muscles. Next you do lunges, again working your legs and buttocks, and then you head to pull-ups, which engage the back and biceps muscles.

Just three bouts each week of intense circuits like this, and you've met the ACSM's requirement for both resistance training and vigorous cardio exercise.

At a minimum, you should perform resistance training and cardio at least once a week. How much you concentrate on each form of exercise depends on your training goals. If you're training for a marathon, you're going to want to do more aerobic-based workouts to build your cardiorespiratory fitness. If you're a power lifter, you're going to concentrate on building strength in the gym. And if your training goal is to stay fit and strong for long-term health, I'd suggest that five workouts a week is the sweet spot. Try aiming for one workout every weekday; inevitably there will be at least one day that's too busy, and so you can do your fifth workout on the weekend. Make sure to switch things up, too. Just lifting weights five times a week will get boring. Try taking a few new classes at a local gym to see what interests you.

WHAT SHOULD I DO FIRST IN A WORKOUT, CARDIO OR WEIGHTS?

When answering this question, consider what you're trying to achieve with your training. The general principle is that your body will adapt to whatever demands you impose upon it and will adapt most strongly to whatever demand is last. So, if you're trying to build your cardiovascular capacity in order to run a faster 10K, it makes sense to do the cardio last, so that your body is geared toward developing aerobic fitness. But if your goal is to amp up your bench press or simply get bigger overall, you'll want to do cardio first and resistance training second. In both cases, it's best to have a goal and develop a strategy for reaching it. That way, you'll get there a lot faster.

If five workouts a week is better than three, why not go for more? What's wrong with six or seven times a week? I often work out all seven mornings in a given week because I crave the stress relief; exercise also sets me up mentally for the day. That said, I'll do something different each day, and not all my workouts are super-intense. Sometimes I'll just do an hour of stretching. The problem with working out hard every day is that you start to get into diminishing-returns territory. The body needs time to recover from its workouts. Six hard workouts a week won't necessarily provide you with additional benefit. It won't improve your cardiovascular system much more than the fifth workout of the week. And a sixth workout won't add to your strength that much. All it's guaranteed to increase is your chance of injury.

Of course, we have to consider real life in all of this; we have only so much time in our days. If you can work out only four times a week, you can feel good about that. Three times a week is the minimum to maintain fitness, but if you don't make that one week, it's not the end of the world—just try to get back into the swing of things the week after.

6

MY DAY WENT SIDEWAYS, AND NOW THE NINETY MINUTES I'D RESERVED FOR EXERCISE HAVE BECOME FIFTEEN. WHAT SHOULD I DO?

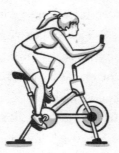

This happens to the best of us. Maybe there's a work emergency. Or perhaps appointments and meetings and your various everyday duties have taken longer than you thought they would. Whatever the case may be, don't despair. Even if you have only fifteen minutes, you can still get in a healthy dose of exercise with a session of high-intensity interval training (HIIT).

One of the world's experts on the benefits of HIIT is McMaster University's Martin Gibala, the author of *The One-Minute Workout: Science Shows a Way to Get Fit That's Smarter, Faster, Shorter*. His studies have shown that, in terms of building aerobic fitness, a HIIT session of sprints and short rest breaks can provide the benefits of a much longer endurance exercise session.

For example, one of Gibala's early studies demonstrated that three short workouts per week on an exercise bicycle, with each session including four to six all-out sprints of just thirty seconds, provided the same aerobic benefits as about four and a half hours of moderate-intensity exercise.

"It's incredible in terms of the physiological benefits that it provides," Gibala says. "You can maintain fitness extremely well with these small doses of intervals through particularly busy work times."

The exact exercises will depend on what you want to get out of your workout, as well as how much time you have. If you're just looking to boost your aerobic capacity—that is, your ability to exercise at a moderate pace for a long period of time—any exercise that features short bursts of all-out activity will help. Just make sure that exercise is something your doctor has cleared you to do—and particularly, that the doctor has cleared you to conduct the sort of intense exercise we're discussing here.

If you *really* don't have much time, one of Gibala's most famous studies showed that even a single minute's worth of hard exercise can provide the same benefits as forty-five minutes of moderate-intensity exercise. In the study, the one minute of all-out exercise was split up into three twenty-second sprints, spaced out over the course of ten minutes.

The sprints in these exercises could be on a stationary bike, but you can get the same benefits from intervals by running up and down stairs. Any activity you can make into an aerobic activity, from running to burpees to body-weight circuit training, will provide similar benefits.

You can also feel free to sprinkle those twenty-second all-out sprints throughout your day. When you have to go up a few floors in your office building to speak with accounting, say, you could sprint up the stairs. Don't walk to the corner store for a bag of milk—strap on your running shoes and sprint! Or if you commute in your car, when you get home, hop on your bicycle and do some sprints as you're tooling around your neighborhood.

Want to get in some strength training as well? Perform sprints with body-weight exercises. Start with thirty seconds of push-ups, then immediately move (without rest) to thirty seconds of air squats. Then leap right into the same duration of pull-ups and repeat.

Gibala's favorite HIIT workout takes him a little over twenty minutes to complete. Though it's not the most time-efficient one out there, this one is simple, easy to remember, and relatively simple to do. He calls it the 10 × 1: one minute of high-intensity exercise followed by one minute of recovery, repeated ten times.

Once you've warmed up, start with a minute of hard cycling at about 85 to 90 percent of your maximal heart rate, followed by one minute's recovery of easy cycling time. (An easy, back-of-the-envelope way to calculate your maximal heart rate is simply to subtract your age from 220.) If you don't have a heart rate monitor, your effort level on the beginning sprints should be around a 5 or 6 out of 10, ramping up to a solid 9 out of 10 by the end. It's better to cycle slowly for your rest interval, rather than stay still, because the easy cycling keeps the blood circulating throughout the body.

Once your minute rest interval is up, sprint for another minute. Repeat the cycle for a total of ten sprint intervals over twenty minutes. Or do less if you really don't have the time. After all, the lion's share of the training stimulus comes with the first interval, with each successive sprint delivering diminishing returns.

Keep in mind that you don't necessarily need an exercise bike to do these intervals. I do mine on a treadmill, and it's possible to increase your heart rate to the necessary level with just about any aerobic exercises, even if it's just sprint jogging in place. So if you're short of time but still craving exercise, plug your earbuds into your ears, put on some heavy metal (or whatever you find inspirational), and let the intervals begin. One suggestion, though: if you're doing them while at work, you might want to close your office door first.

WHAT'S THE BEST WAY TO
MAINTAIN STRONG BONES?

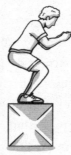

Anything that bashes and puts an accelerative force on the bones will help keep them strong. One person who knows about the practical side of bone strength and weakness is Timothy Kopra, a US Army colonel and astronaut who has spent 244 days in space over two missions and served as the commander of the International Space Station.

The rough rule of thumb for astronauts is that without exercise they lose about 2 percent of their bone strength for each month that they're in space. Exercise is intended to mitigate the effects of weightlessness; however, one survey of thirteen astronauts found that even if they did exercise, their bone strength decreased by an average of 14 percent during their six-month missions on the ISS. That decrease in bone strength then puts them at greater risk of breaking their hips later in life, when they're back on Earth.

Astronauts on the space station have three basic options for exercise in the zero-gravity conditions of orbit. The most important one for protecting their bones is a weight machine known as the Advanced Resistive Exercise Device (ARED), which is designed to allow space station personnel to do any number of different resistance-based exercises. The ARED is equipped with springs and other motion dampeners to ensure that the inertial effects of weight lifting don't damage the space station. Thankfully that's not a concern on Earth, where it's just as important for us terrestrial civilians to exercise regularly to maintain bone strength.

Osteoporosis, a disease in which the bones grow brittle and more susceptible to breaking, is something that was historically associated with women. But bone strength can be an issue in men, too. One in three women will get osteoporosis, and the condition will affect one in five men. More than 80 percent of fractures that happen after the age of 50 are the result of osteoporosis.

According to Osteoporosis Canada, peak bone mass exists between the ages of 16 and 20 in women and 20 to 25 in men. Even young adult and middle-aged men lose a little bone mineral density each year—somewhere between 0.4 and 1.5 percent annually. One estimate says that if men were tested for bone mineral density, a third of those over 65 would be prescribed calcium and vitamin D supplements, to build bone strength.

But supplement-based therapies have their problems. Side effects exist, and then there's the cost. Exercise-based therapies may be more practical. They're certainly cheaper. But what sort of exercise is best?

Any physical movement that stresses the bones will strengthen them. It's a mechanism that comes from evolution—an action creates a stress on the body, and the body responds by changing itself to prepare for the next instance of the stress. In the case of a jarring or compressive force on the skeleton, the body interprets the force as a signal that it needs stronger bones to decrease the risk of injury the next time around, so it activates biological processes that make bones stronger.

One way to exert force on the bones is through resistance training that targets the major muscle groups—squats, bent-over rows, dead lifts, military and bench presses, lunges, and calf raises. For people at risk of osteoporosis, resistance training of the major muscle groups twice a week is a good baseline.

Jumping is another alternative. Scientific studies have shown that jumping of all sorts—from one-legged hopping to two-footed squat jumps, forward hops, zigzag bounding, and hurdles—can build bone strength. You don't want to start by leaping into the air from a platform, though. Begin with easy jumps that start and end with you on the ground. As you gain confidence and strength, mix it up. Or don't: studies have found benefits for both schoolchildren and adults who did as little as performing a set of ten jumps where they simply leaped up as high as they could into the air.

Running can also provide you with the jarring impacts required to increase bone strength. In fact, a British study of pre- and post-menopausal women found that as little as one minute of running was enough to strengthen bones. Interestingly, the pace required to increase bone strength in the subjects fell with age. That is, the premenopausal women had to run fast to get the proper effect, while postmenopausal women were able to strengthen their bones with just a slow jog.

Regardless of whether you're lifting weights, jumping, or running quickly—or using an Advanced Resistive Exercise Device while orbiting the earth—jarring or compressive force on your bones is what keeps them strong. As to which sort of exercise you choose, it's up to you: your bones aren't fussy.

ARE THERE ALTERNATIVES TO YOGA FOR IMPROVING FLEXIBILITY?

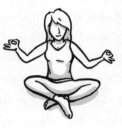

Yes, of course. But before we start talking about alternatives to yoga, I want to make sure you understand its benefits and have at least given it a shot.

Some people hear the word *yoga* and summon up an image of an activity that just isn't for them. They envision a stereotypical yoga practitioner who is into spiritual practices, burns incense, loves organic food, and prefers alternative Eastern medical techniques such as acupuncture to Western medicine. (Not that there's anything wrong with any of those things!) All the same, that perception doesn't apply anymore.

Before I began doing yoga about ten years ago, I felt it wasn't for me. Then I found a great instructor, Laurie Campbell, who sold me on the benefits of the practice.

I like several things about Laurie's classes. One, they're intense, so I feel as though I'm getting a workout. Two, she's open-minded and practical about physical activity, and she views yoga as a tool that helps the body exercise in a healthy, sustainable way.

"I don't necessarily think people should just do yoga," she says.

"I think people should *move*. If people are moving, and they're doing it at a high intensity or high frequency, then they should also *recover*—which is where yoga comes in."

Physically, yoga promotes core strength and flexibility. In other words, people who do yoga are able to move better, with fewer injuries. But yoga also provides a mental benefit: it relieves stress, and its meditative components promote personal well-being.

I am not someone who is naturally gifted at yoga. My muscles don't seem willing to stretch. No one would ever feature me in a YouTube video showing how to perform a sun salutation or a warrior pose. For years, you would find me on the mat, my muscles shaking, sweat dripping from my brow, as I pushed myself into one pose or another.

But yoga helped me slow down. My natural pace tends to be *go, go, go*. Yoga forces me to collect myself. Yoga is also humbling. It isn't a contest, and no one cares how good you are at it.

So even if you feel as though yoga isn't your bag, I would suggest you try it out. Start by going to one of the better-established studios in your area because they tend to feature classes for beginners. Bigger studios also provide mats for a small rental fee, so you don't even have to make that investment. If you've never done a class before, you might feel silly and self-conscious the first couple of times you go. But doing something you've never done before is good for you. And you'll quickly discover that no one's judging you.

Don't stop with your first class, even if you hate it. In fact, I'd challenge you to attend six classes before you decide whether you're going to pursue yoga. With each class, you'll feel less self-conscious. Going into classes three and four, you'll find that you're better able to get your body into the poses. Feel silly assuming the more pretzel-like positions? Approach it from the point of view of a child: try to access your inner sense of play.

A large part of yoga focuses on breathing. There's a meditative appeal in the flow from pose to pose—and the challenge when you're just beginning is that you're so intently concentrating on what the instructor is saying that you're not able to focus on the breathing. It takes most people until classes five and six to be able to start grasping the calmness and pleasure in the human body's movement that can come from a really good yoga session.

The other thing about giving yourself half a dozen classes before you decide whether to pursue yoga is that it provides you with an opportunity to try out different teachers. Some instructors talk a lot. Others are silent between their directions. Some like ambient music; others, hip-hop. Some provide lots of direction to students when a pose may not be just right. Others prefer that their students learn poses on their own. What you like comes down to personal preference.

DOES STATIC STRETCHING PREVENT INJURY DURING EXERCISE?

Gym teachers, coaches, personal trainers—for ages they've been telling us we should push ourselves into all sorts of uncomfortable positions to limber up our muscles before we exercise. And as a society, we've subscribed to the practice, doing everything from quad pulls before a spell of cycling to prerun standing toe touches. Experts call this static stretching—slowly pushing into a position that elongates a particular muscle for up to thirty seconds at a time.

We stretch for a number of different reasons. Some of us do it because we believe it'll prevent injury. Others stretch to avoid soreness *after* the activity. And still others do it because they believe they'll get better performance from their muscles.

However, well-designed scientific studies have demonstrated

that static stretching doesn't usually achieve what we think it does. With an obvious interest in the topic, USA Track & Field conducted a study that followed 2,700 people for three months. Half of them stretched before workouts, half didn't. The result? No significant difference in the injury rates between the two groups.

When it came to soreness, a similarly designed study out of Australia found that people who engaged in static stretching were less likely to experience exercise-related muscle soreness—but only by a tiny bit. Another study, out of Texas, found that stretching actually *reduced* the maximum strength of a given muscle.

What's it all mean? Think of a muscle like an elastic band; over-stretching it can reduce its ability to store energy, reducing the power and strength of its spring.

That's a risk with static stretching, at least. *Dynamic* stretching, on the other hand, is designed to get the blood flowing through muscles and warm up the body, and it continues to be recommended in preparation for strenuous physical activity. Jumping jacks, walking lunges, and the groin-stretch movement that audiences see hockey goalies perform during a pregame warm-up are all forms of dynamic stretches. So if you're preparing for some athletic activity, consider eschewing those long, painful static stretches for more fun and effective dynamic warm-ups.

If, after six classes, you still feel that yoga isn't for you, then first, I offer my congratulations. Good for you for trying something new. Then I would direct you to the numerous different classes and alternative forms of flexibility training that are appearing in major cities across the continent.

Essentrics is a form of flexibility training that features elements of ballet and tai chi. Ido Portal is an Israeli movement coach whose teaching, known as "ido," combines elements of yoga as well as gymnastics, capoeira, and martial arts, and who has worked with the MMA fighter Conor McGregor. Tai chi may be beneficial to maintain flexibility and range of motion.

And in many major cities, you'll find new studios solely devoted to stretching, such as LA's Stretchlab, New York's Power Stretch Studios, or Stretch Zone, which has dozens of locations across the United States.

"People look up to elite athletes," Laurie Campbell says. "They want to *train* like elite athletes. But many of those athletes perform yoga to recover from their training. Everyone needs to complement what they do with something else."

If you're serious about your training, it makes sense to regularly do some form of activity designed to ensure that you maintain your range of motion and minimize the possibility of injury. For many people, that complementary session is yoga. But if you've given yoga a shot and decided that it's not for you, you still have many alternative options that will provide similar benefits.

9

WHAT THE HECK IS $VO_{2\,MAX}$, AND WHY ARE EXERCISE PEOPLE OBSESSED WITH IT?

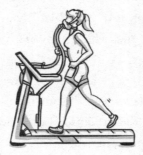

$VO_{2\,max}$ is an abbreviation that represents a person's maximal oxygen uptake—basically, it's the rate at which your body can transport the oxygen that is used as fuel in the mitochondria of your muscle cells. The faster your body gets oxygen to those mitochondria—and the more oxygen it delivers—the faster and longer your muscles can operate.

Basically, then, your $VO_{2\,max}$ is a measure of your cardiorespiratory fitness. If you get out of breath climbing a flight of stairs, you likely have a low $VO_{2\,max}$; conversely, if you can cycle up hills with no change in your breathing, your $VO_{2\,max}$ is likely sky high. But $VO_{2\,max}$ measures a lot more than just your fitness level; it also functions as a useful indicator of your risk of dying from cardiovascular disease and other causes. In 2016, the American Heart Association issued a statement that called on health professionals to consider using $VO_{2\,max}$ as a vital sign—that is, as an indicator of one's overall health—along with more traditional risk factors, such as blood pressure and resting heart rate.

What is so special about $VO_{2\,max}$? Maybe the most important thing is how many different parts of the body influence it. Not only is it affected by the ability of the lungs to get oxygen out of the air and into the blood, but another factor is the arterial blood vessels' ability to transport that oxygenated blood to the muscles, which, in itself, depends on the heart's capacity to pump the blood. It's also determined by the ability of muscle mitochondria to convert oxygen and fuel into energy that is then used by muscles to create movement.

Stressing the cardiorespiratory system, whether by brisk walking, jogging, cycling, or working an elliptical machine at the gym, signals to the body that it should improve itself. The muscles grow more mitochondria to burn fuel. The heart grows bigger and stronger to improve its pumping capacity. The blood vessels relax, increasing their interior diameter and allowing more blood to flow through—a property known as "endothelial function." All of that improves your $VO_{2\,max}$.

The better an athlete you are, the better your $VO_{2\,max}$ is, especially in endurance sports. For reference, at rest, the body has an uptake of 3.5 milliliters (ml) of oxygen per kilogram (kg) of body weight per minute. The average North American 40-year-old male has a maximal oxygen uptake of 35 to 38 ml/kg per minute; the average female, 31 to 33.

Genetics accounts for about 50 percent of your $VO_{2\,max}$, but training can improve your score. The highest most of us can get with training is a bit over 60 ml/kg per minute for men and the lower 50s for women. (The highest-ever $VO_{2\,max}$ score published in academic literature is 90.6 ml/kg per minute, registered by an Olympic champion cross-country skier.)

I had my $VO_{2\,max}$ assessed last year. It took about fifteen minutes on a treadmill adjusted to give the impression of progressively steeper climbs, the better to tax my cardiorespiratory system. While I exerted myself, I wore a breathing mask connected to a device that measured the difference in the oxygen contents of the air I inhaled and exhaled.

It was one of the toughest medical tests I've ever done. But I'm glad I did it. The evidence shows that a relatively small increase in your fitness—an improvement of just 3.5 ml/kg per minute—is equivalent to losing more than two and a half inches of waist circumference, in terms of reducing your risk of dying from cardiovascular disease. In fact, many would argue that as an indication of your overall health, your $VO_{2\,max}$ is as good as better-known metrics such as blood pressure or resting heart rate.

So why is it so difficult to get a $VO_{2\,max}$ score? Right now, $VO_{2\,max}$ tests aren't a regular part of clinical practice. That's partially a reflection of the equipment required, which few doctors' offices have. I think it also has something to do with the medical profession's reluctance to champion the health benefits of exercise.

Wouldn't it be nice if you could get your $VO_{2\,max}$ assessed at your local pharmacy or gym? The machine could be in the back, by the blood pressure monitor. Many universities will provide you with a $VO_{2\,max}$ score for a fee. The rest of the medical profession will catch up, one of these days. And when it does, we'll all be healthier for it.

10

IS IT OKAY TO SIT ALL DAY IF I
GET IN MY DAILY WORKOUT?

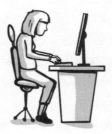

This is a question that's becoming more and more pressing every day. Research during the last few years indicates that sitting is an independent risk factor for all sorts of health problems, even for people who work out daily.

That's a problem, because many of us sit more than we do anything else. We sit in the car or the commuter train as we head into work. At the office, we sit at our computers and in the conference room. Historically speaking, human beings may sit more now than they ever have. Decades ago, we might have stood up from a desk to go and speak in person to a work colleague on another floor. Today we simply send that person a text message or email. And when we finish work and go home, many of us plop down on the couch and sit for another several hours as we stream the latest TV series.

The conventional wisdom long suggested that all that sitting is okay as long as we've gotten our daily dose of physical activity—a fitness class, an hour in the bike saddle, or a good 10K run.

Then, back in 2009, new findings detonated that thinking. Tim Church was one of those researchers. The professor of preventive medicine at Pennington Biomedical Research Center at Louisiana State University was among a group who wondered whether sedentary behavior had any effect on our overall longevity. To discover the answer, Church and his fellow scientists looked at a Canadian survey, the 1981 Canada Fitness Survey, which included about 17,000 adult men and women.

For the survey, researchers visited people in their homes and asked them about such daily habits as whether they smoked, their alcohol consumption, and their leisure-time physical activity levels. Separately from all that—and the reason the survey was pretty unusual—they were asked to estimate the amount of time per day that they spent sitting during work, school, and housework. Then the researchers followed the men and women for thirteen years, tracking their health throughout the study period, noting who died, who lived, who stayed in good health, and who contracted disease.

Church and the team discovered a troubling association between how much people sat and how long they lived. Essentially, the longer they sat per day, the sooner they died. Put another way, time spent sitting was positively associated with the risk of dying from all causes, including cardiovascular disease. Later studies have confirmed the conclusion, linking prolonged periods of sitting with greater risk of diabetes, depression, and obesity.

The key finding in all this, however, was that the risk of dying prematurely was higher independent of how physically active the subjects were. It didn't matter whether they jogged, worked out at a gym, or swam—the amount of time they spent sitting still affected their risk of dying prematurely.

Why is sitting so bad? Scientists don't yet have an answer for that, but they speculate that a lot of different factors are at play. Long periods of inactivity may reduce the amount of blood that can be pumped through the heart. The end effect is to increase the risk of cardiovascular disease and type 2 diabetes. The takeaway here is that exercising does not cancel out the effects of sitting.

So what to do?

I wouldn't bother trying to convince your boss to shell out thousands of dollars on an expensive ergonomic chair. "The people suffering from neck and low back pain, related to sitting, they get one of these fancy ergonomic chairs and they *still* have neck and low back pain," says Dr. Andrew Miners, a chiropractor who is the director of sports medicine at Medcan. "The problem isn't that they're sitting in a bad chair; the problem is that they are sitting too darn long."

To ward off sitting's ill effects on health, use motion to break up prolonged sedentary periods. Fidget, in other words. As someone who finds it difficult to keep still for long periods, I like that advice. I'll stand up and walk around during meetings to get the blood flowing in my legs. If you are chained to your desk by a deadline, consider using a standing desk or sitting on an exercise ball. It also may help to take a short walk around the office, or around the block, once an hour. And if you're at home, relaxing with some TV, get up and walk around at least once an episode. Better yet, perform exercises such as crunches or push-ups every so often through the show. The idea is to move every moment you can.

Sitting can also harm your posture. To prevent that, consider a quick bout of stretching.

"Sitting is a *flex* posture," Dr. Miners says. "When you're sitting at your computer, everything is bent or curled over. Your back is hunched, your neck is craned down, your *fingers* are even bent."

To change things up, every so often, perform a motion that is the *opposite* of sitting—what Dr. Miners calls a standing extension relief. To demonstrate, he stands up tall, as though he's being pulled by a rope from the top of his head. Then he arches his back, inhales deeply to expand his thoracic cage, angles his head as high as his neck allows, and extends his arms out as widely as possible.

To avoid the health risks of sitting for long periods, the advice comes down to a pretty simple takeaway: Don't sit for long periods. Break up the sedentary periods in your work and your leisure time with motion, whether a bit of fidgeting or a full-body stretch. Your later-life self will thank you.

11

SHOULD I EXERCISE HUNGRY
OR AFTER EATING?

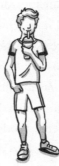

Physiologists refer to your state of hunger as either *fed* or *fasted*. Whether you should conduct your physical activity fed or fasted depends, like a lot of things having to do with exercise, on what you're trying to do. Are you trying to lose weight? Get healthy? Improve your aerobic fitness and thus your ability to run endurance races? Or build muscle mass and size?

Let's tackle muscle mass first. After a strength-training workout, two competing processes are happening in the muscle tissue. The training has prompted the creation of new muscle protein. But at the same time, some of your existing muscle protein has broken down as a result of the stress of the training. The trick is to try to synthesize, or create, new muscle protein faster, and for a longer period of time, than the old protein breaks down.

Though protein *breakdown* isn't much affected by the fed or fasted state of the person exercising, protein *synthesis* is. That's why body-builders down protein shakes during and after their workouts—to get their muscle tissue into the fed state, providing it with the dose of protein needed to boost protein synthesis. So if you're trying to build muscle and strength, exercising in the fed state helps.

If you're concentrating on endurance exercise—running, cycling, doing your cardio on an elliptical—you may want to exercise *fasted*, possibly first thing in the morning. Why? Research shows that physical activity in the fasted state tends to burn more fat. However, there are some trade-offs to consider before you make your decision.

One of the more famous studies to illustrate the fat-burning benefits of exercising fasted was published in 2010 by a Belgian-led team. They wanted to re-create an environment in which people eat too much high-fat, calorie-dense food, such as end-of-year holidays or a summer vacation. The members of one test group consumed a high-fat, high-calorie diet but exercised in a fasted state each morning before they ate breakfast and drank only water during the exercise. Those in another group consumed the same diet but did their morning exercise in a fed state, after they ate breakfast. They also consumed a sugary energy drink during the exercise. All told, both groups exercised four times a week: twice running, twice cycling. A third group consumed the same diet but didn't do any exercise.

After six weeks, the results were pretty remarkable. Those in the control group, who hadn't exercised, had gained an average of more than 6 pounds in the six weeks that they consumed the high-calorie diet. Those in the group that exercised after breakfast, while quaffing the sugary drink, gained a little more than 3 pounds. And those in the group that exercised before breakfast, in a fasted state, didn't gain weight at all. They also managed to avoid losing their insulin sensitivity, an important health marker, while the members of the group that exercised in the fed state and drank the sugary drink lost their insulin sensitivity—a significant stepping-stone toward type

2 diabetes. That study, and others like it, show that exercising in a fasted state and consuming only water during the exercise is a more effective weight control strategy than exercising full.

HOW DO YOU KNOW WHETHER YOU'RE HYDRATING PROPERLY?

Drinking enough water is key to optimal training and racing. Because different people sweat at different rates, it's tricky to specify exactly how much any individual should drink in absolute terms. One important sign of proper hydration is a moist mouth—if your mouth feels like a desert, you're probably dehydrated. Having to urinate every ninety minutes to two hours is a good sign that you're hydrating properly, as is the color of your output: your urine should be a light yellow color when you're properly hydrated.

The theory is that when working out aerobically, such as running or cycling, the body tends to burn carbs first to fuel its performance. If the body has carbs available to burn, that's what it will use. But if there aren't many carbs available—which can happen first thing in the morning if one hasn't eaten since dinner the previous night—the muscles use the next best thing available: fat.

Finally, what if you're concerned about performance? There, too, is evidence that things will improve if you train in a fasted state. Research conducted in Australia and Canada, among other places, has shown that conducting a few weeks of training in a carbohydrate-depleted state can boost all sorts of performance adaptations, including the ability to burn fat for energy. The research has led to the concept of "train low, compete high"—that is, train when your carbohydrates are low, but, come race day, provide your muscle cells with all the carbs they need to work at their highest function by ingesting energy drinks, as well as gel packs and energy bars.

Bear in mind, though, that the benefits of this "train low, compete high" approach are controversial. Take Medcan registered dietitian Rachel Hannah, an elite runner who won bronze in the marathon at the 2015 Pan American Games and who is busily training in the hope that she'll represent Canada in the marathon at the 2020 Summer Olympics in Tokyo. She cautions that training in a state of depleted carbs can feel terrible—so bad that it can prevent the athlete from training as hard as possible, which in turn can blunt the performance benefits of training. "My main goal right now is staying healthy and performing at a world-class level," she says. "Every session matters for quality, and I don't want to sacrifice the quality of the session by trying to do it fasted."

Training fasted also may leave you more susceptible to illness or injury. That's why exercise physiologists suggest conducting only *some* training sessions in the fasted state. Tossing in a week or two of carb-depleted training, in which muscle cells must switch to burning fat stores for energy, is believed to provide those same cells with the ability to perform even better when their carb levels are high.

You can also use a range of techniques during carb-depleted training to fool your body into working hard. Taking a dose of caffeine is one example, as is swishing a carb-loaded energy drink in the mouth, then spitting it out, which some studies have shown provides athletes with the ability to train harder.

So when making the decision whether to eat breakfast before a training session, consider your goal. If you're trying to build muscle, go ahead and eat protein before, during, and after the training. If you're looking to burn fat, exercise fasted. And if it's performance gains in an endurance race that you're after, feel free to experiment.

Training fasted just may make your muscle cells feel supercharged when they finally have all the carbs they need during the race.

HOW TO EAT TO RACE

The following are the types of foods that Rachel Hannah prefers before, during, and after a big event. When you're planning your big day, use this menu as a model.

Before

Soy milk with coffee

Oatmeal with a banana and a little nut butter (peanut, sunflower seed, or almond)

Yogurt

Half a banana ninety minutes before the race and a single gel pack about ten minutes before the start

During

An energy drink every hour, mixed to a concentration that provides between 50 and 60 grams of carbs per hydration

After

Whey-based protein drink

High-protein snack bar

Peanut butter or almond butter sandwich

Yogurt with fruit and nuts

Cottage cheese and a piece of fruit

Hummus and baby carrots with a piece of fruit

Hard-boiled egg with whole-grain crackers and hummus

12

WHAT'S THE FASTEST WAY TO GET INTO THE BEST SHAPE POSSIBLE?

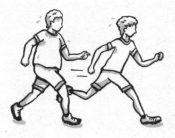

Like most of us, I've faced a lot of situations in my life where I had to get into great shape fast. When I was in college, it was the return of rugby season. Later in my life, a group of friends and I vowed to climb Mount Rainier near Seattle. Only about half the people who attempt to summit the mountain make it to the top. The run-up to the climb coincided with a period of intense work, and in the weeks beforehand, I worried that I was going to be one of the people forced to turn back because I was out of shape. Maybe you've been in a similar situation, worrying about your fitness as you head toward some kind of a running or cycling event.

The good news is that it's possible to get into great shape quickly. As long as you're healthy and cleared by your doctor for intense exercise, you just have to work hard. Before we get to that, however, I want to preface all this by saying that getting fit doesn't have to be so difficult. It's a fun and enjoyable experience for most, particularly if you begin training five or six months before your big event.

The following method is more of a Plan B in case you haven't had the time to train properly, maybe because an injury or travel got in the way.

One of the world's experts on $VO_{2\,max}$ is Michael Joyner, a professor of anesthesiology at the Mayo Clinic College of Medicine in Rochester, Minnesota. Joyner is fascinated with something called the Hickson Protocol, which he's identified as the fitness regimen that boosted subjects' cardiorespiratory fitness faster and in a shorter amount of time than anything before or since.

The Hickson Protocol was designed for a study conducted at Washington University in St. Louis, Missouri, that required eight subjects to exercise for forty minutes a day, six days a week, for ten weeks. The protocol had the subjects alternate between interval training days and days of hard running at a steady pace. On their interval days, they pedaled on an exercise bike in six sets of five-minute intervals, separated by two minutes of rest. On the long run days, they ran as far as they could in forty minutes—that is, they set off and raced as fast as they could for forty minutes. During both types of training, what was most important was the pace. The five-minute bike intervals took place at $VO_{2\,max}$ pace—basically, the subjects cranked the pedals almost as hard as they could.

The results paid off. The subjects' $VO_{2\,max}$ increased by an average of 44 percent. Four of the subjects attained $VO_{2\,max}$ levels of 60 ml/kg per minute, far above the average $VO_{2\,max}$ for American 20-year-old males of 43.2 ml/kg per minute. By the end of the study, the subjects were in the top 5 percent for their age group. Basically, Dr. Joyner says, "these people went from kind of an underperforming clunker to a higher-end Lexus."

Joyner believes that the most effective part of the subjects' training was the long, hard intervals. So to give your fitness the quickest boost, do workouts that utilize this HIIT approach. Each interval should be somewhere between three and five minutes at a time, going as hard as you can. Don't bother trying to do more than six sets—it's doubtful that you'll want to, anyway.

HOW LOW CAN YOU GO?

Many people wonder about the minimum commitment required to stay in the best shape possible. The question is of special interest to time-pressed professionals. I go through periods where I'm in great shape, and then I'll hit a period of intense time demands. That's when my focus becomes doing the minimum required to avoid losing the fitness I've acquired.

After Hickson established the training regimen that boosted his subjects' fitness so quickly, he began investigating the minimum effort required to *keep* superfit people in such impressive shape. That is, now that they were fit, how little could they do and still *stay* fit? What he discovered is that it doesn't take much effort to stay in shape, as long as you're willing and able to exercise hard.

To prove this, he took a group of subjects and ran them through ten weeks of the Hickson Protocol. Then he split the group in half. One group reduced its training by one-third. The other group reduced its training by two-thirds—those in the group that was exercising the least ran or cycled for just thirteen minutes a day, six days a week. On their interval days, they performed only two intervals of five minutes each on an exercise bike. And on their running days, they ran as hard as they could, but for just thirteen minutes.

By several different measures of fitness, including $VO_{2\,max}$, heart rate, blood lactate threshold, and body weight, the group with the lower duration of training retained their benefits. The only fitness measure that decreased was the amount of time it took for them to get fatigued on a long-term endurance test, and that decreased by only 10 percent.

"The key factor was the intensity," Dr. Joyner says. "I could see this working for busy executives who want to follow a program when they're on the road, so that when they get back, they're ready to go."

Hickson's results show, then, that most people will be able to retain their fitness with a two-thirds reduction in training duration, as long as they keep incorporating high-intensity intervals into their fitness routines.

Plotted on a graph over time, the Hickson Protocol's per week increase in $VO_{2\,max}$ shows a steep, straight line of improvement. The subjects in the Washington University study followed the protocol for ten weeks, but Hickson couldn't convince them to continue their training past that—the workouts were just too tough.

Feel free to pursue the same approach over a shorter duration if that's all the time you have. Want to get into the best shape possible in just two weeks? Do the Hickson Protocol for two weeks. Have longer than ten weeks? Theoretically, the fitness-boosting benefits may continue—although Dr. Joyner expects that for most people, the increase in fitness will level off once males reach a $VO_{2\,max}$ in the high 50s or low 60s, and females reach the low 50s.

13

CAN I TAKE A PAINKILLER BEFORE
MY EXERCISE SESSION?

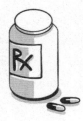

I've run a number of marathons, and of them all, I found New York to be the toughest. I'd never considered Manhattan to be terribly hilly, but that day it seemed to be—so much so that I bonked at the end of the race.

It had never occurred to me that I could have taken ibuprofen before the race to tamp down the pain. If I'd been paying more attention, I would have noticed that the practice is becoming increasingly common among cyclists, marathoners, and ultramarathoners.

The idea is that if you pop an ibuprofen or two before a long race, you'll be better able to handle the discomfort that comes when you're trying to push against the limits of your body. If you take pain out of the equation, you can register a better time.

I understand the thinking. But the practice isn't wise.

The best athletes stay in touch with their bodies. Muscles, ligaments, fuel stores—they all provide signals to the brain, and elite athletes stay aware of those signals, the better to determine whether it's possible to push the body to a faster pace or to ease off a bit because an injury is ahead.

Painkiller use blunts the relationship between brain and body, and it can make injury more likely.

"If you find yourself taking an ibuprofen to satisfy a fitness goal, you need to step back for a moment and realize that you may have reached a point where your quest for fitness may be undermining your long-term health," says Chris Mear, a Medcan fitness trainer.

I agree. Sometimes exercise hurts, but most of us are adept at distinguishing the good kind of hurt—the one that comes from a hard but healthy workout—from the bad kind that leads to injury. Some types of fitness gyms and trainers celebrate those who push this line. A few years ago, adherents of one particularly intense form of fitness training lampooned this type of boundary pushing in the form of cartoons of "Uncle Rhabdo," a muscular clown afflicted with rhabdomyolysis—a potentially fatal condition that happens only in the most extreme cases of overly strenuous workouts. Damaged muscle cells die and eject their proteins into the blood, the muscles swell, and in extreme cases a surgeon must slice open the skin to relieve the swelling. Though it's extremely rare, "rhabdo," as it's known, is no laughing matter. No responsible trainer would ever push a client to that extent.

Many of us are under the impression that physical performance and health increase proportionally to each other. The better or more strenuously an athlete performs, the healthier we tend to think that athlete is. But the people who achieve the most impressive performances may actually be sacrificing their long-term health in any number of ways. Think of the long-retired football players whose knee injuries become evident when they toddle out onto the field during NFL games, the former pro tennis players with back or shoulder problems, the runners who incur joint issues thanks to repetitive stress.

The best kind of exercise is fun. Mind clearing. Stress relieving. If you're getting to a point where you're regularly taking ibuprofen to train harder or race harder, you might consider examining your whole attitude toward fitness.

The practice of taking a painkiller before exercise may not make scientific sense, either. A 2017 study conducted by Stanford University's Baxter Laboratory for Stem Cell Biology, based on experiments in mice, suggested that exposing muscle tissue to the class of painkiller to which ibuprofen belongs—known as nonsteroidal anti-inflammatory drugs (NSAIDs)—harms muscles' ability to recover from training.

There's a cycle to muscle regeneration: Training damages the muscle tissue, activating pathways within the body that then repair the tissue and make it stronger than it was before. Some of those pathways also happen to involve pain and inflammation, and NSAIDs blunt those pathways. The medication prevents the pain and inflammation—but it may also prevent the repair cycle that improves muscles' exercise capacity. At the cellular level, no pain means no gain.

So what if you've done your training and you just want to pop the painkiller for a race in order to snag a personal best?

That situation is also risky. One 2017 Stanford University study of ultramarathoners found that 44 percent of the runners experienced kidney injury after fifty miles of running. Those who had taken ibuprofen before they ran the race were 18 percent more likely to experience the injury—and the injury they experienced was more severe. (The study's lead author said he believed that the racers' kidneys returned to normal in the days after the races.)

Regardless of whether you're training to build strength or endurance, it seems clear that you shouldn't use painkillers as a way to train harder, because they may prevent your muscles from adapting and growing stronger due to the exercise. The issue is a little less clear for taking painkillers during a race. The risk of a temporary injury to the kidneys is higher; that seems clear. But some people may decide that the short-term damage is worth it to try to achieve a personal result. Just don't fool yourself into thinking that such a race is improving your health. It's ironic, but sometimes the long endurance events that people run to prove their fitness just might prove unhealthy in the long term.

14

I USED TO LOVE EXERCISING, BUT NOW I CAN'T FIND THE MOTIVATION. WHAT SHOULD I DO?

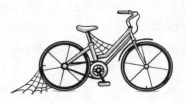

Though it would be nice to think that you can just pick up a book, read about how great fitness is, and then set off on a course for weekly workouts that you will follow for the rest of your life, that's not the way humans work. At some point you're going to get bored with the way you're exercising. Everyone does. That's fine. It's what you do next that's important: you don't quit. Here are five tips to keep that from happening.

MAKE YOURSELF ACCOUNTABLE TO SOMEONE

One thing that will help keep you consistent with your exercise is creating a supportive team to help motivate you. "You've got to find something that will make you do it when you don't want to do it," says Greg Wells, an exercise physiologist at the University of Toronto and the author of *The Ripple Effect: Sleep Better, Move Better, Eat Better, Think Better*. He describes a hypothetical situation that will sound familiar to many people. His example is a 55-year-old woman, an accountant, who has just had a brutal day. "She gets home from work, and she sits down on her couch and she's like, 'I'm done, I'm going to watch TV.' "

What's going to get that woman off the couch? What's powerful enough to give her the energy or the motivation to get to that exercise class? Wells likes the idea of training with a partner. Find a friend to go to the gym with you. Sign up for a running group. Join the collection of enthusiasts who populate CrossFit gyms. Or join a sports team.

It isn't important who it is. What's important is that you're going to do better with someone.

CHANGE YOUR GOAL (OR SET ONE)

Let's say you've been running for a while, and you're bored. Consider signing up for a race. When it comes to races, start small. Sign up for a 5K and resolve to walk it briskly. The point of your first race is to put yourself in a positive situation, heading down a route demarcated by supporters on either side clapping and holding signs for people like you. That experience can provide you with exactly the inspiration you need to reinvigorate your fitness. And if the 5K seems too easy? Good for you—make it a 10K, a half marathon, or even an ultramarathon. It doesn't matter what it is—just make it *something*.

Perhaps you don't want to participate in a competitive event. The Color Run is an untimed 5K that bills itself as the "Happiest 5K on the Planet." It involves participants' beginning in white shirts and being sprayed with colored powder all along the course, followed by a party celebrating everyone's achievement. Or you could sign up for a noncompetitive obstacle course race, such as a Tough Mudder. Whatever it is, a goal can work wonders to get you up off the couch and into your exercise clothes.

CHANGE HOW YOU'RE WORKING OUT

Maybe you're bored by the way you're working out. Let's say running's not doing it for you anymore. So don't run. In fact, move as fast as you possibly can *away* from running. Switch things up.

"Here's the base formula: there is no base formula," says Dr. Tim Church, the director of preventive medicine research at the Pennington Biomedical Research Center at Louisiana State University. "There is no right way [to exercise]. The right way is what works for you. Some people say, 'I hate exercising in the morning.' So don't exercise in the morning. There is no best way; the best way is the way that keeps you doing it."

Your exercise time is too important to waste on something you don't like. So if running's getting stale, try cycling or swimming, or sign up for a spinning class. Take up yoga or Pilates. Any activity is better than none.

CHANGE HOW YOU THINK ABOUT WORKING OUT

Make your fitness social. Take advantage of the numerous options for free and outdoor fitness classes or groups available in most every city. Friends can gather together for workout sessions. After-work exercise classes can even end with glasses of wine and conversation that wouldn't be out of place in a bar. Some of the classes are free.

For too long we've considered exercise a chore. It's time to evolve our thinking past that. Set up appointments with friends to participate in an exercise class. What you'll find is that over time, exercising evolves from a chore into the highlight of your day.

TAKE A FITNESS VACATION

If you're feeling uninspired and bored by the notion of any exercise at all, commit to a vacation that requires some minimum level of physical fitness. Perhaps it's a hiking trip in a national park or a yoga retreat. Maybe it's a more exotic, bigger trip—a cycling tour of French vineyards, a walking tour of Peru, trekking in Nepal, or a summit bid for Mount Kilimanjaro. Whatever it is, nothing is going to motivate you to get out of bed more than the thought of a vacation several calendar pages away. Just make sure you make the vacation realistic and achievable. Exercise is too important to feel guilty about it.

15

SHOULD I INVEST IN A FANCY
NEW FITNESS WEARABLE?

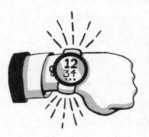

Yes, if you think it'll help you. With names such as Fitbit Flex, Withings Pulse, and Polar Loop, and app-ready devices such as the Apple Watch, high-tech methods to monitor the healthfulness of your lifestyle are exploding. Fitness monitors and apps are a booming industry.

The good news about fitness trackers is that they're relatively good at what they do. If your activity tracker says that you took 8,421 steps on Monday, you likely came pretty darn close.

But statistical accuracy isn't necessarily the reason that so many people are buying such trackers. We're buying them because we want them to help us. If we're sedentary, we want them to help us get moving. And if we're already fit, we want them to help us become *more* fit.

Among the lowest tech of the trackers is a pedometer, a simple device worn on your body that tallies each step that you take. Some studies have shown that just the simple act of tracking this information can motivate you to increase the number of steps you take in a day. Higher-tech devices have been shown to be even more effective than simple pedometers at increasing the amount of exercise you get. The likely reason? The apps have been engineered to make fitness fun.

The data from such devices are also helping researchers understand the way people move. For years, physical activity data relied on surveys and simple devices to determine how people move about in the world. Sometimes researchers worried that the data weren't very accurate. But the devices being sold today, with their miniature accelerometers and heart rate monitors (among other sensors), are providing researchers with a detail of real-world information never before seen.

For example, in 2017, researchers at Stanford released an important study that tracked people's physical activity based on information collected from smartphones. The data set was enormous, a total of 68 million days of "minute-by-minute step recordings." The results revealed that users in forty-six countries around the world get an average of about 5,000 steps per day. They also pointed out how important the "built environment" is to people's likelihood to walk. The city where people walked the least was Jakarta, the Indonesian capital, home to 10 million, where only 7 percent of the roads have sidewalks. In fact, Indonesia came last among the forty-six countries in terms of step counts, with just 3,513 steps taken per day on average. The highest? Hong Kong with 6,880, followed by China with 6,189.

Another revealing finding was that the walkability of a given city affects people's tendency to be physically active, suggesting that investments in urban infrastructure designed to promote walking, such as wider sidewalks, may promote people's health and decrease obesity rates.

It's important to realize that smartphone apps and fitness-tracking devices are not only monitoring your activity levels; they're also tracking how you use them, with a view to making you more likely to use them. That's good, because data show that most people get bored with trackers and apps over time.

"The mind tends to wander," says Dr. I-Min Lee, the Harvard epidemiologist. "Once people become familiar with something, they're less likely to be interested in it. So you have to keep changing things."

Fitness trackers will improve as the technology matures. Stephen Lake is a cofounder of Thalmic Labs in Ontario, Canada, which develops new ways for humans to interact with technology, such as an armband that controls a computer. "Imagine you're going for a run," says Lake. "And a display floats ahead of you in your field of view." The display might feature your pace and your heart rate. Or it might show the point where your next hard interval will start. Or it could display messages from your friends, "people giving you kudos for exercising as you're exercising," says Lake. "Which would gameify exercise, changing it into more of a social activity."

That's a few years off, however. Today, if you think a fitness wearable or app will help make you more physically active, go for it. But don't let the fact that you don't have one keep you from working out.

16

WHAT'S THE BEST EXERCISE TO IMPROVE MY MOOD AND MENTAL HEALTH?

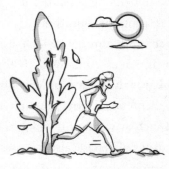

Most people who exercise regularly will be able to recount a story about the way exercise helped lift them out of a bad mood. Or how it enabled them to break through a seemingly intractable situation. Or just simply brightened their day. I can be as irritable as I've ever been, and all I need to do is go for a run or a bike ride, and my grumpiness lifts. I think part of it is the fact that it's tough to feel bad about the world when you're on a running trail or out for a good ride. The world is a beautiful place, and sometimes it takes a bout of outdoor exercise to encourage that realization.

Studies have shown that exercise can improve alertness, allay anxiety, and improve depression. Some researchers have claimed that exercise can be as effective as medication in treating certain aspects of mental health.

In fact, some physicians and psychologists believe physical activity is a much better prescription than medication. It can take weeks and even months for a clinician to determine the proper dosage of an antidepressant, which can cause such side effects as weight gain, dry mouth, nausea, fatigue, and decreased sex drive. Exercise, in contrast, can elevate your mood after the first bout of activity. And its side effects tend to be more positive: improved sleep, improved self-image, possible weight loss, and even a strengthened sex drive. It may not solve the underlying issue, but it is a cheap, healthy, and immediate way of treating the symptoms.

The exact mechanism through which exercise does this isn't known. One theory is that exerting the body through physical activity can spur neuron growth in the hippocampus, a part of the brain that is affected by depression. Strenuous physical activity releases neurotransmitters, such as serotonin, which is central to the action of antidepressant drugs. Exercise also releases endorphins, which give the so-called runner's high euphoria that can follow a bout of physical activity.

But what if you want the *most* elevation in mood? What exercise is best? That depends on whether you're talking long term or short term. Over the long term I'm going to give you one of those non-answers that so often comes out of the mouths of exercise experts: the kind of exercise that will most elevate your spirits is the one that you're most likely to do. Because over the long term, it's the *frequency* of exercise that is the most effective way to maintain your spirits. Yoga, endurance training (running or cycling), indoor circuit training classes, strength-boosting resistance sessions—all of them have been shown to boost mood and fight depression. And each one has its own particular benefits. Yoga seems to be better at fighting stress. Resistance training may tire you out, leading to better sleep. Sustained aerobic exercise can also introduce mental clarity to your thinking. The point? Do the one that you enjoy the most at the moment.

In the short term, again, you kind of have to go with your gut. I prefer a tough high-intensity interval training workout—something vigorous that's run by an upbeat, encouraging trainer in a fitness studio with some great music; something that has me giving everything I have for a short amount of time, that gets me out of my head and gives me some distance from whatever was bugging me, followed by a rest, where all I can do is concentrate on getting my breath back.

Exercise may be the last thing you want to do when you're down. But there are very few things that are as effective at creating a short-term elevation in mood. I believe in the power of physical activity to treat numerous human problems—including a cloudy disposition. So if you're feeling low, consider donning your workout clothes and engaging in your favorite physical activity. The exertion may not eliminate the problem that provoked the gloom in the first place. But your mood is bound to be better than it was before your workout.

Part Three

THINK

HOW CAN I MAKE THE
CHOICE TO BE HAPPY?

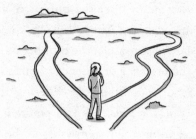

It goes without saying that happiness is one of the most important foundations for good health. The first step toward long-term happiness is recognizing that happiness is, in large part, a choice. That might be hard to believe, but there's research to back it up.

Shawn Achor is the author of *The Happiness Advantage: The Seven Principles of Positive Psychology That Fuel Success and Performance at Work*, which discusses the challenge of staying positive and productive in a difficult world. His theories are based on the way the brain constructs a picture of reality. According to Achor, that basically amounts to a data management problem.

At any one time, we can perceive potentially hundreds, if not thousands, of things about the world around us. What we perceive is important, because it not only allows us to form plans but also influences our emotions.

Say you're a pedestrian attempting to cross an intersection during the noon-hour rush. Your data-gathering tools—your eyes and ears and, to a lesser extent, your nose—harvest tremendous amounts of information about the world around you. There's the color of the traffic light across the street and the fact that the other pedestrians around you are waiting for the light to turn green. There's the sound of cars passing in front of you. All of those data suggest that you, too, should stay still and wait on the corner. And so you do.

But how does your brain filter the important factors from all the other information available? After all, it's possible you also take in the color of a bystander's trousers, the number of taxicabs parked across the street, or the presence or absence of birds in the sky.

According to Achor, our brains are filtering the information that's necessary to us *all the time*. "As you perceive the world," he says, "your brain is scanning a few snowflakes in the midst of a blizzard."

The decision whether or not to cross the street involves short-term filtering. But we also conduct long-term filtering. Throughout the course of a day, week, month, and year, we're deciding where to place our focus, where to exert the energy required to store our memories, and how to frame the recollection of an experience. Let's say that I've just finished saying good-bye to the guests we invited for my son's birthday. How do I frame the event in my mind? Do I focus on that awkward moment when I couldn't remember the name of my boy's best friend's mom? Obsess over the fact that he cried when everyone looked at him to blow out the candles on his cake?

Or do I think about the happiness in my boy's eyes when he opened his gifts? And the delight he experienced when he took in the trick conducted by the party's magician?

One of Achor's main points is that the brain is constantly deciding what to notice and what to disregard. "We take in only a small fraction of what's happening," he says. "It's our choice what we take in."

Achor's thesis is that a person's happiness is only loosely predicted by one's external circumstances. According to Achor, who studied under the happiness guru Tal Ben-Shahar, only 10 percent of one's happiness is dictated by the external environment. The rest—the other 90 percent—is predicted by the way your brain processes your circumstances.

Knowing that, is it possible to change the way one perceives and processes reality? Absolutely, says Achor. In fact, it's important that we do. Many people in industrialized societies have a flawed relationship with happiness. We think that happiness is something we achieve when we get something—when we land a great new job, win a big deal, or achieve a personal best in a race.

But often, Achor says, the reverse is true. You don't become happy because you've achieved success; rather, you achieve success *because* you're happy. That's what he calls "the happiness advantage."

I can see many people screwing up their faces and shaking their heads as they read this. It sounds silly, doesn't it? It's so against the grain of the way those of us in North America think about the state of being happy. But it's true—it is possible to *become* happy. To train our brains to register our experiences in a way that improves our perception of well-being. To essentially *rewire* our brains.

Happiness is crucial to our performance in any number of ways. Achor calls happiness "the fuel that turns on the brain to its highest possible level." Citing academic studies, he says that a happy brain performs 31 percent better than a brain that is negative, neutral, or stressed. Or take job performance: whether or not one is successful in one's career is dictated by one's intelligence, but only up to 25 percent. The rest of one's success comes from social factors—whether you have strong social supports and, more important, how you perceive the world and whether you view stress as a challenge. In other words, whether you're *happy*.

So how can you train yourself to become happy? Many different techniques exist. Achor has combed the psychology research and compiled a few of the easiest and most effective. One strategy is to write down, every day for twenty-one days, three things for which you're grateful. Another is to create a habit of writing about a positive experience you've had in a journal each day. A third is to develop a habit of writing an email or letter expressing gratitude to someone every day.

Get the idea? Each of the above encourages you to fix a positive memory in the brain. In so doing, the brain crowds out negative ones.

"It's not necessarily reality that shapes us," Achor says. "But the lens through which you perceive reality."

There are lots of ways to increase one's short-term happiness. But over the longer term, Achor's "count one's blessings" techniques may be just enough to nudge you out of a morose outlook toward a more positive one.

DO I NEED THERAPY?

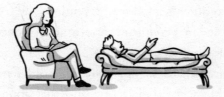

That's a question that only you can answer. But one thing is certain: more people would benefit from some form of mental health treatment than are getting it.

It's common for athletes, when they're healthy and doing well, to consult with high-performance coaches in an effort to perform even better. The trouble is, very few people approach their mental health similarly. That's too bad.

The way that society thinks of counselling is similar to what dominates in the medical world, where the emphasis is on curing disease and treating symptoms rather than promoting the health of unique individuals. To me a more rational model is a preventive approach in which the emphasis is on the promotion of optimum performance.

How does that approach look in practice?

Ideally, we would all work to promote our mental health in numerous ways. That means not just engaging in self-care strategies such as sleeping enough, eating well, and exercising regularly but also regularly checking in with mental health professionals.

"Many people wait until things are really dire before reaching out to a professional for help," says Gina Di Giulio, a Medcan psychologist. "While it is important to seek support when one is unwell, a preventive approach to therapy is best." The idea, she says, is that "it's easier to put out a small flame than a fire."

A proactive approach to therapy might take several different forms, says psychologist Mike Friedman. "I think the 'check in' approach every so often is good for prevention," he says. "You're feeling iffy, you come in a couple of times and get things squared away before a full-blown problem emerges."

Performance enhancement is something different, in Friedman's mind. Rather than occasional check-ins, that approach would require ongoing coaching. That relationship might be more like an arrangement with a personal trainer or a music instructor. You would set a goal—say, overcoming the shyness that afflicts you in social situations. Then, through regular sessions, you would create a strategy to meet the goal.

"If you're serious about performance enhancement," Friedman says, "you generally want to be doing regular sessions in some capacity to keep your progress on track."

Throughout my life, I've benefited from the advice of numerous different types of advisers, from performance coaches to psychologists to life coaches. One of the most effective forms of ongoing mental health maintenance that I've found is regular sessions of group therapy. A handful of my peers and I get together regularly and, in a nonjudgmental, confidential, and supportive way, discuss any issues we're facing—personal, professional, social, you name it. Our group is run through a professional organization, but the same approach could be adopted by anyone.

Others prefer the sort of arrangement that exists with a one-on-one relationship with a mental health professional, whether a psychologist, a performance coach, or some other form of therapist.

Mental health professionals are happy to work with clients in a preventive capacity. Known as "booster" or "tune-up" sessions, the typical model sees a client who is not struggling with any particular malady or issue checking in every so often. For example, one of Di Giulio's clients schedules a quarterly appointment with her that coincides with his employer's quarterly performance review. He just knows, when his review is up, that it's time to see his psychologist, regardless of what is happening in his life.

"We book annual physicals for ourselves," Di Giulio says. "It makes sense to do the same for our mental health as well."

There are many ways to find a professional who is a good fit for your personality. Your general practitioner will happily provide you with a referral. If you don't have a GP, you can get a referral from an outpatient clinic. Religious leaders, friends, and family also may be able to provide useful suggestions, and you can come up with names of qualified professionals by doing online searches or calling such organizations as the American Psychological Association, the Canadian Psychological Association, or the Canadian Association of Cognitive and Behavioural Therapies.

If possible, try to talk to a few candidates before you settle on the one you'll work with over the long-term. "It's a lot of trial and error," says Friedman. "People can do some research on the Internet. You might have a friend who knows a therapist. But ultimately you have to go and see someone. Give it a few chances before you find someone who feels right."

Be prepared for some misses before you get a hit. Hiring a mental health professional isn't the same as hiring an auto mechanic. Only you can decide whether you might benefit from therapy, and if you think you will, it's important to have a good rapport with the person who is doing the listening.

3

IF WILLPOWER IS A MUSCLE,
HOW CAN I EXERCISE IT?

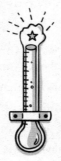

Science has shown us that willpower is a resource that can be exhausted and strengthened. The strength of a person's willpower fluctuates throughout a day. It starts strong, in the morning, just like the body's physical muscles, and then decreases as you exert it. For example, let's say I have a task that requires focus, like the writing of this chapter. What might take me an hour in the morning, when I'm focused and disciplined, is apt to require three hours if I have to do it at night, when I'm tired.

The most famous research into the science of willpower is the series of "marshmallow experiments" conducted at Stanford University in the 1960s and early '70s, which presented kids with a conundrum: the researcher set a marshmallow before a child and said it was fine to eat the marshmallow immediately. However, if the child waited a few minutes to eat the snack, the researcher would reward the child with an extra marshmallow. About a third of the 600 kids in the first experiment waited long enough to be awarded the second marshmallow.

The researchers followed the kids over time, and it turned out that the ones who had displayed better self-control during the study performed better in school. Subsequent experiments have established that self-control is one of the few quantifiable human qualities that corresponds to greater success in life. People with more self-control tend to do better in their careers, have lower rates of drug abuse, enjoy deeper relationships with other people, and even weigh less.

The best-known figure in the science of willpower is Roy Baumeister, the social psychologist who literally wrote the book on the topic, together with the science writer John Tierney. Baumeister's research has contributed to the understanding that willpower is an expendable resource. Each decision that you make represents a decrease in the amount of the resource available to you.

One great example of the expending of willpower is the action of staying focused on a single task on a computer. Early in the day, when your store of willpower is high, it's a relatively simple matter to reject the impulse to go off task, check a sports score, or investigate a sudden manifestation of your curiosity.

Let's say I'm editing a speech that I have to give at an upcoming event. I head to a website to research the executive introducing me. But then another item—a story about the fifty most influential people in Toronto—catches my eye. Should I go see whether I recognize anyone in the list?

This time, I decide to stay on task. But the more frequently I resist temptation, the less willpower that I have to make the same kind of decision the next time around.

The more choices you make, the more willpower you use up. And the less willpower you have, the poorer your decision making becomes. That leads to some fascinating dodges. People with low stores of willpower are more likely to try to avoid making a decision. They'll postpone the mental effort required, figure out some way to skip doing so altogether, or default to the status quo. One thing that they *don't* do, Baumeister says, is compromise—because compromise requires a complex mental calculation that taxes the will. "When you're depleted from exerting self-control, you tend to simplify the task and make a very simplistic sort of decision," he explained in an interview with *Barking Up the Wrong Tree*, a science-based blog about success.

I try to schedule my days so that I do the difficult, important stuff first. If a tough decision comes up late in the day, I'll try to put it off until the following morning, when my store of willpower is strongest.

Another way that some people apply this? They limit their wardrobe options. President Barack Obama used this principle by wearing only blue or black suits. The idea is that choosing what to wear is a decision that one makes early in the morning, when willpower stores are high. In order to conserve their decision-making ability for more important choices, some people—the late Steve Jobs was famous for this—wear the same thing every day.

If you feel as though your store of willpower is depleted, one effective way of bolstering it is by eating something. Baumeister's lab employs sweet snacks, which work well if you need to boost your self-control only in the short term. If you require greater self-control over a longer period of time, a protein-laden snack is better. Another tactic is to get some rest. Taking naps tends to be problematic at work, though, so consider adjusting your nightly schedule so you get more sleep.

"Rest is good," Baumeister says in the online interview. "The longer people have been awake, the more self-control problems happen. Most things go bad in the evening. Diets are broken at the evening snack, not at breakfast or in the middle of the morning."

Another tactic when faced with a difficult decision is to think of a role model, one who has demonstrated excellent willpower and who can inspire you to exert greater self-control yourself.

Once you understand that willpower and self-discipline are like muscles, it becomes reasonable to start exercising them, the same way one might train a biceps or pectoral muscle. Research has shown that exercising willpower in small, simple steps builds your self-control for other things down the road. Take the kids in the marsh-mallow experiment: choosing to wait for a second marshmallow might have decreased their store of willpower in the short term, but if they had repeated the experiment on a daily basis, it might have strengthened their willpower, giving them more self-control when faced with other temptations.

All signs point to willpower being a mental muscle. Happily, that means that many of the tactics designed to strengthen it are similar to what would strengthen any other muscle in your body: ensure that your blood sugar level is at an optimum level, sleep well and sufficiently, and exercise in small, simple ways to strengthen your discipline for bigger decisions.

4

I'M SO STRESSED OUT THAT I CAN'T WORK
PRODUCTIVELY. WHAT SHOULD I DO?

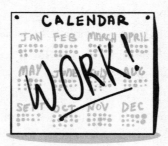

There is a short-term and a long-term answer to this question. The short-term answer, according to Dr. David Posen, an MD, stress expert, and the author of *Is Work Killing You?: A Doctor's Prescription for Treating Workplace Stress*, is that you should stop what you're doing, take a break, and go outside. Things will look a bit better once you've cleared your head.

The long-term answer is more complex. "So many people are setting themselves up for this kind of thing," Dr. Posen says. "They're trying to do too much. Their expectations are totally unrealistic. After forty or fifty hours a week, productivity falls off pretty dramatically. If you're so stressed you can't work productively, your body is giving you a message—you need to slow down."

Some people can't slow down, however, because they're slammed in an unavoidable extended period of intense work—what Dr. Posen calls a "work blitz." One person who can speak to the phenomenon of the work blitz is David Urban. He's an impressive guy—a West

Point grad who won a Bronze Star serving with the 101st Airborne Division during Operation Desert Storm, who has gone on to become a respected Republican political operative, the owner of a major Washington lobbying firm, and a frequent talking head on CNN. During the last US presidential election, he found himself running the Republican campaign in Pennsylvania—which meant stress, and lots of it, for months at a time.

But you don't have to be managing a presidential campaign in a key battleground state to feel stressed out. Many of us experience prolonged periods of stress. The classic example Dr. Posen uses is the demand blitz that happens to accountants at tax season. Another example is retailers during the holidays. I've also seen this happen to the staff of a start-up that's prepping for a round of investment seeking. Stress can come in numerous forms. But it doesn't have to defeat you.

One strategy he suggests to prepare for an extended work blitz is to catch up on your sleep. "Make sure you're well rested before you start," he says. "Next, clear the decks. Anything that is extraneous, anything that can be set aside—set it aside."

The third thing he suggests is, if it's at all possible, to pace yourself. "You must have one day a week where you can step away from all of it," he says. "Your body and your mind have to recover."

One of the key things Urban does during campaigns to keep himself sharp is to cut out alcohol and caffeine. Why? Because, he says, using them can develop into a vicious spiral. You wake up exhausted, mainline caffeine to get an edge throughout the day, then turn to alcohol in the evening as a way to relax. But that cycle prevents you from sleeping well, and then you wake up tired (or hungover) the next morning—which in turn requires more caffeine to get you going.

"When you're getting pounded by stress every day," Urban says, "you can get in a vicious Ping-Pong cycle with caffeine and alcohol. So cutting out any kind of stimulants or depressives is extremely helpful."

The key to managing stress is to avoid that out-of-control feeling that sees you flitting from crisis to crisis. To avoid that, institute a daily routine. Sleep is important. No matter what hotel room happens to be home that evening, when Urban is in campaign mode, he tries to go to bed and get up at the same times each day. He has an order to his morning that sees him taking some time first thing after he wakes to read the newspapers before opening his email inbox. And he tries to exercise, regardless of whether it's in an actual gym or just a hotel workout room.

"When I was in the military, going to the gym was part of your job," Urban says. "In the corporate world, people want you to be fit and healthy and on top of your game, but then they give you a certain look when you're heading out to the gym. It's up to you to build that into your life. Make it a priority. That's not being selfish—that exercise is part of your work."

There's no right or wrong setup. What matters is that you establish a routine and stick to it, because that routine is the thing that will help you manage the demands on your time and keep stress at bay.

Finally, remember that every stressful period is temporary. Whether it's election night, the moment a deal closes, or the day you finish a big project, there is always an end. If things feel unbearable, look forward to the time when they'll become incrementally more bearable.

So if you start to feel things getting out of hand, eliminate from your life the things that add to your stress, such as the cycle of alcohol and coffee. Try to maintain a routine that includes adequate sleep and exercise. And in those moments when you just don't know whether you can handle things, remind yourself that the situation is temporary, that the stress has a conclusion. And if you can't see that end point? Figure out a way to create a finish line and visualize the steps along the way that will take you there.

5

WHAT'S THE MOST EFFICIENT WAY
TO MAKE A GOOD DECISION?

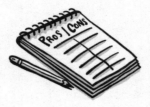

How can we make good decisions? Social scientists, psychologists, and economists have been exploring that issue at least since the eighteenth century, when an English statistician, philosopher, and Presbyterian minister, Thomas Bayes, began theorizing about event probability, a key factor in making decisions. Studies during the centuries that followed established the way that biases affect our ability to make good decisions.

In his book *Thinking, Fast and Slow*, the Nobel Prize–winning psychologist Daniel Kahneman refers to the *planning fallacy*—the human inclination to be too optimistic when considering the possible benefits and costs of future events. The planning fallacy is why contractors are apt to provide one estimate for a kitchen renovation and then, months later, invoice for a much higher price.

Also playing a role in human decision mechanics is what Kahneman refers to as *loss aversion*—a behavioral tic that biases our actions toward avoiding losses rather than pursuing gains. The bias is so powerful that psychological research once suggested that a gain needs to be twice as large as the potential loss for humans to pursue a gamble.

In 2007, a team of UCLA psychologists studied the reward circuitry in the brains of people who were considering whether to take a financial risk. As loss aversion predicted, the reward circuitry reacted more to losses than possible gains. But what was fascinating was the way the reaction depended on whose brain was being studied. That is, the UCLA team found that different people exhibit different amounts of loss aversion—which in turn explains why some people are more comfortable than others with taking risks.

The question, then, is whether there's a way to nullify the effects of our various preprogrammed biases so that we make the best decisions possible. Absolutely, is the answer. In fact, your friendly neighborhood library likely has several shelves of books that provide guidance on how to do just that.

One of the better guides to making a great decision is by David Welch, a political scientist now at the University of Waterloo. In his 2001 book *Decisions, Decisions: The Art of Effective Decision Making*, he describes a simple, step-by-step plan for how to consistently make the best choice in any situation.

The first step involves identifying the objective. This is likely the simplest part of the process. We face a variety of decisions throughout the day: what shirt to wear; whether to take the subway, drive the car, or ride a bike to work; which assignment to work on first.

The second step involves determining options. Sometimes this involves a lengthy list, like at a restaurant where many different menu choices exist. Other times, it's a simple binary choice between two things.

The third step is to examine the decision's implications. Picking

TAKING A MOMENT TO REFLECT

When I have something important to mull over—a major, life-changing decision—I like to head away from the city to somewhere quiet. It could be a cabin in the woods, a town in the countryside—anywhere I can get away from the "noise" of daily living and the demands of technology. My thinking happens on long walks that see hours go by without any intrusion.

Such personal retreats are a great way to do the really deep thinking required to make the best decisions. So when you have an important life-changing choice to make, take the steps required to give it the attention it deserves. Giving yourself the uninterrupted time required to determine the best course of action may just require getting away from it all.

an item from the restaurant menu is pretty inconsequential to anyone but you, but deciding how best to save for your kids' education or whether to buy a new home can have major ramifications for the lives of you and your loved ones.

The fourth step is assessing the import of your decision. That is, how much is the decision worth agonizing over? Daily living requires us to make lots of decisions, most of which aren't all that important. Try to reserve your mental energy for the really consequential stuff. On this matter I like to apply a version of the "80/20 rule": 80 percent of your mental energy should be devoted to the most important 20 percent of your decisions.

After those four steps, Welch suggests that the next part of the process is budgeting for the time and energy you'd need to make the decision. Then comes the part when you actually formulate a decision-making strategy.

That last part, in particular, is key. Decide how you're going to make the decision. Compare the benefits versus the costs—more complex decisions may require more complex strategies. Consider the decision to buy a car, for example. In that case, you might develop a formula that sees you scoring various cars based on the satisfaction you get from them, then dividing each car's score by its cost. Just like that, you've created a ranking of the vehicle's "units of satisfaction per dollar."

"Decision making has elements of art," Welch acknowledges. "It cannot be reduced to a certain technical exercise." That's true, but if you follow Welch's advice, you can make your decision-making process more efficient. Establish your objective, consider your options, and weigh the implications of each possible choice. Then, based on importance, set a time and energy budget for the decision. Doing that will help you determine the strategy for how you'll make the call. Once you have that lined up, make your choice—and don't look back.

6

HOW CAN I GET OUT OF THIS
TERRIBLE RUT I'M IN?

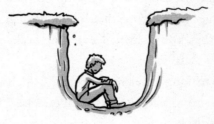

My trainer, Thomas Adriaens, is one of the most consistently enthusiastic people I know. I'll head out for a session with him, usually on my bike, and he'll never be anything less than in a great mood. It's not a facade—he's genuine. I once asked him how he does it. He shrugged and answered me in his charming French accent: "I love my job."

It's hard for me to imagine, but there was a time when he wasn't so enthusiastic about his job. Years ago, Thomas had a career in finance, but one day, he realized that work was weighing him down. Inspiration? That irrepressible French *joie de vivre*? Neither of those was possible when his life revolved around numbers on a spreadsheet. He wanted to be outside, working in a way that would exhaust him physically. He wanted to change people's lives. So he became a personal trainer.

Several decades later, Thomas's customers contract his services on a per appointment basis. Every time someone hires him for an hourlong training session, he tells himself, it could be his last. He needs to be enthusiastic and engaged so that the client wants to hire him again. Basically, his incentive structure is perfectly set up to ensure that he stays motivated and inspired; if he's not, he'll be out of a job.

Most everybody, at some point in their lives, feels uninspired by their career or some other element of the day-to-day. And if you feel as though you're in a rut, you may not be able to make the sort of large-scale career change that worked so well for Thomas.

One of the best ways to combat that feeling is to ensure you have something to anticipate, something that makes you feel hopeful and provides your life with a spark. Maybe it's a new relationship. Joining a new sports team. A special vacation with your child, or parent. Or maybe it's a new project at work. Whatever it is, that excitement tends to brighten every other part of your life. And if you have more than one thing that inspires you, your life is all the better for it.

So if your goal is to be as enthusiastic as Thomas each day, you have to ask a question: How can I go about changing my life?

I've been experimenting with the potential of microhabits. That's a philosophy that suggests that a series of small, incremental changes can translate into substantive transformation over time.

For example, a new microhabit I recently developed was going without sugar in my coffee. And that's changed my life—honestly, it has. I can hear a skeptic saying that that sounds like nonsense. How can opting for unsweetened coffee transform one's life?

Here's how: I'm eating better. I've lost some weight, which is making me feel faster on my bike. I'm happier when I put on my clothes, because my clothes are fitting better. Not only that: the sugar rush I used to get from my coffee elevated my energy levels early in the morning—and then crashed them at a key point, right when I was getting to work. Now that I'm going without the sugar rush, I'm more even-keeled just as I get to work, which sets me on a better path throughout the day.

I see microhabits as one achievable way to improve your life. Make them easy to do—remember, they're *micro*habits. They're tiny changes to your everyday routine that add up to improve something bigger.

For example, one of my friends started setting out her running outfit each night, before she went to bed. She took her top, tights, socks, and running shoes and set them out in another room so that when she woke up, she could steal out of her sheets in the morning silently, without waking her partner. Suddenly she was running five mornings a week rather than just one or two.

A colleague of mine stopped setting his cell phone on his nightstand. Instead he kept it in the kitchen, which was on the same floor but far enough away from his bedroom that he wouldn't be tempted to check it before he fell asleep. The tiny change meant that he fell asleep a good half hour before he used to, which was just enough to get him recharged and invigorated for work each morning.

Another colleague started limiting himself to two drinks when he went out with his friends for their weekly Thursday-night get-together. That got him home at a decent hour, rather than last call, which in turn meant he had more energy for the Friday-night date night he had with his wife each week.

Everyone is apt to fall into a rut once in a while. Sometimes getting out of a rut requires a major decision: making a career change;

taking that adventurous trip you've been considering; moving to a new city—or even a new country. But try establishing a new micro-habit before you do something drastic. Little changes can trigger major transformations—ones that may even be enough to pull you out of the rut you're in.

7

CAN I LEARN HOW TO BE OPTIMISTIC?

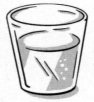

It's entirely possible to learn how to be an optimist. But don't limit yourself to just becoming optimistic. What *kind* of optimistic person you become is just as important.

The conventional way to think about optimism and pessimism is to consider them as innate character traits—features that are fixed, that we can't change. The classic differential presents a person with a cup of water. Does the subject say it's half full or half empty? The answer is supposed to reflect the subject's innate positivity or negativity. The half-full optimist will tend to believe that events will turn out fine, while the half-empty pessimist is apt to believe that somehow, some way, things will end badly.

But recently, some psychologists have posited that it's possible to change this character trait. It's a way of thinking called *positive psychology*, described by University of Pennsylvania professor Martin Seligman in his book *Learned Optimism: How to Change Your Mind and Your Life*. Positive psychology aims to improve personal well-being rather than cure already developed maladies.

Seligman's theory targets the cause-and-effect linkages that we create when considering our personal histories. Let's say a pessimist fails a math test. He's likely to ascribe the failure to the fact that he's just not intelligent enough, while an optimist would say the failure was the result of not enough studying. See the difference? The pessimist believes his failure was due to an innate quality that can't be changed; the optimist chalks it up to lack of work and resolves to do better next time. One path leads the pessimist to reduced horizons, while the other triggers improvement that may spur the optimist to a better result the next time around. So an optimistic, taking-responsibility-for-one's-successes-and-failures approach is a good way to think about the narrative of one's life.

Things are a little different when considering future events. Being optimistic about achieving a goal isn't enough to make you successful. Rather, a certain subset of optimistic thinking is what helps.

Psychologists have grouped the way pessimists and optimists think about goals into three categories. According to a paper written by New York University psychologist Gabriele Oettingen and her coauthors, pessimists use a technique called *dwelling*, which means "reflecting on the present reality possibly standing in the way of one's desired future."

Let's say a runner has a race a few days away, and he or she is considering whether to set a goal to qualify for the Boston Marathon. If the runner is a pessimist, he or she is likely to dwell on all the things that could go wrong: "I could be late to the starting line. I could twist my ankle in a pothole. I could bonk around mile twenty." The pessimist's "dwelling on" strategy makes it difficult to achieve goals. Focusing on all the things that could go wrong discourages the pessimist from expending the effort that is required for success.

Optimists pursue one of two strategies. Some do something that

Oettingen calls "indulging": they fantasize about meeting their goal and all the good things that are apt to happen because of their success. What they don't do, however, is consider what it will realistically take to get there.

The same marathoner, as an indulging optimist, might see himself crossing the finish line, arms raised, under the time required to run the Boston Marathon. Perhaps he sees himself later wearing a T-shirt from the marathon or describing the race to another, less gifted, envious runner. But those are all future successes; the strategy of indulging isn't an effective way to motivate action in the present, which means that indulging doesn't correlate with success.

The other optimistic approach, which Oettingen's team calls the "most effective route to goal pursuit" is called "mental contrasting with implementation intentions." Effectively, it's a combination of indulging and dwelling. It's the linking of "a critical situational cue to a specific goal-directed behavior"—what psychologists describe as "*if* obstacle, *then* goal-directed action."

To engage in mental contrasting, you need to spend time visualizing the positive outcome of an event. You also need to consider all the things that could go wrong along the way. The difference from just dwelling on the negatives is that you think through the various steps required to overcome the obstacles. You make plans. You prepare.

For example:

"*If* there's a chance I could be late to the starting line, *then* I'll leave an hour earlier, to give myself a buffer."

"*If* I'm worried about stepping in a pothole, *then* I'll watch the ground as I run."

"*If* there's a chance of bonking in the race's final miles, *then* I'll take along the water and carbs required to fuel my body."

Ultimately, the optimist's most effective goal attainment strategy involves setting a goal, visualizing potential obstacles, and then thinking through plans to surmount those obstacles.

The method has both physical and mental benefits. Adults who were taught mental contrasting were twice as physically active as those who used other strategies. Students who used the strategy while preparing for their SATs were likely to study more, and when Oettingen's team taught the technique to economically disadvantaged schoolchildren, the children improved their grades, attendance, and in-school behavior.

Qualities such as pessimism and optimism are not ingrained in our characters; rather, we can train ourselves to be more optimistic, chronicling our histories and creating future goals in a manner that increases our chances for success. To do that, take wishful thoughts about a goal and transform them into plans that neutralize obstacles and set the stage for success.

8

IS THERE A WAY TO GET THE BENEFITS OF MEDITATING WITHOUT ACTUALLY MEDITATING?

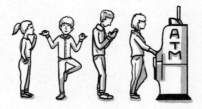

According to a recent study, somewhere around 8 percent of people in the United States use meditation as a complementary health approach. I am not one of them because, well, look, I'm just going to come right out and say it: I find meditating boring.

I know that's sort of the point. But the thought of sitting in a room somewhere, concentrating on my breathing, just fills me with anxiety about the 19 billion other, more productive things I should be doing as those seconds and minutes tick by.

Too bad for me, because mindfulness meditation has a lot of benefits. The practice involves stepping back from the day-to-day bustle and attempting to still one's consciousness. The mindfulness expert Jon Kabat-Zinn, a professor at the University of Massachusetts Medical School and one of the pioneers of mindfulness-based stress reduction, describes it as paying attention to the moment in a way that is simultaneously accepting and nonjudgmental.

A 2011 study out of Harvard Medical School found that eight weeks of a mindfulness-based stress reduction program increased the size of the parts of the brain that deal with learning, memory, and emotion regulation. Other studies have shown that mindfulness exercises can help people cope with stress and anxiety. Those who meditate tend to experience more happiness and an improved quality of life. The practice has also been shown to help people deal with chronic pain.

One basic mindfulness meditation technique is to concentrate on your breathing for a period of time, anywhere from a few minutes to an hour. There are many apps that can provide guidance, and mindfulness coaches and meditation teachers are easily accessible in most major cities.

The benefits are so great that the founder of the Optimal Living Lab, Reva Seth, published a 2017 op-ed suggesting that the Canadian government create a program that encourages the general public to meditate—something not unlike ParticipACTION, the public health initiative that tried to sell people on the values of exercise. "It's time for public-health officials, policy makers and the public to get behind a commitment to scaling up access to meditation," she wrote.

I'm not arguing with Seth about the benefits of meditation. The problem, for me, is that I just can't get around to doing it. What I *can* get behind is combining my meditation with exercise. I get on my bike or lace up my sneakers and head out for a run, and I lose myself in the exertion, the repetitive motion, and my music.

Dr. David Levy, the CEO of EHE in New York, does something similar. Every morning, his dogs get him up and he does one of three things: he goes for a 10K run, a long ride on his bicycle, or a swim.

"When I come to the office in the morning, I have way more clarity of thought than most," he says. "Exercise gives me the opportunity, before the day begins, to have an hour of total mental clarity."

Start by leaving your phone and electronic training devices at home so that you're immersed in the present during your session. The meditative state never happens immediately. You have to find a rhythm first. Once you've found your cadence, sink into it. Imagine that your lungs are bellows, and focus on nothing but your breathing. You'll find that slowly your thoughts will still and your consciousness will almost dissolve.

The exercise doesn't have to be limited to running, biking, or swimming. You can achieve the same effect while sculling on water, jumping rope in a gym, or even hitting a tennis ball against a wall. The whip of the wrist, the upward trajectory of the ball, the arc of its descent—all those things can have a calming effect as your mind loses itself in the moment.

One caution: if you're going to try to achieve this Zen state through exercise, rather than through restful breathing or yoga, you need to have built up your capacity for cardiorespiratory fitness to such an extent that you can run or cycle—or whatever the exercise may be—for a sustained period with comparatively little effort.

The good news is that whether you get your moment of peace from sitting motionless in a room or during a vigorous activity, the boost is the same. There's a calm that lingers for the rest of the day. Irritation, anger, frustration—those states are slower to come on days when you've experienced a calm moment of mindful reflection.

So if meditation is one of those things you think is good in concept but for which you can never find the time, consider leaving your devices at home the next time you head out for a run or a bike ride. Focus on your breathing, establish a rhythm, and give yourself over to the moment. Before long, you'll find that you're sinking into a Zen state that provides the benefits of mindful meditation without the inactivity.

9

WHAT'S THE MOST CONSTRUCTIVE
WAY TO PROVIDE CRITICISM?

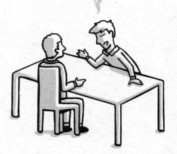

I am both a CEO and a father of three sons. My success in both roles is contingent on the skill with which I'm able to deliver criticism. I have to offer it in such a way that my sons—and my employees—listen to me. They need to respect my opinion to such an extent that they carry out the change I'm asking of them.

When I approach situations that require me to provide constructive feedback, I think about the advice I once heard from Caroline Ouellette, a veteran of the Canadian national women's ice hockey team and one of the most successful hockey players on the planet—she's won four Olympic gold medals, six world championships, and NCAA women's hockey championships as both a player and a coach. In that time, she has played and worked under some of the most successful coaches in women's hockey. Thanks to such mentoring, she has come to recognize several things that are important when successfully providing criticism.

First, she says, "it's easy to accept feedback from someone who leads by example." That is, if a comment is designed to stop an athlete from being late to practice, the feedback will be received a lot better if the coach tends to be reliably early. In the same way, if I'm talking to one of my kids about making his bed, I'm going to be a lot more effective if I, too, am unfailingly consistent in making my own bed.

Second, she says, it's important to be honest, direct, and timely with the advice. She experienced the benefits of this approach toward the end of her career playing with the Canadian women's national team. A few months before the 2014 Winter Olympic Games in Sochi, the coaches called her in for a meeting.

Ouellette was thirty-four at the time, older than virtually all of her teammates. Despite her age, she felt as fit as she'd ever been, and she was confident about her ability to contribute to the team. But during the meeting, the coaches broke it to her that she wouldn't be playing on the first line. In fact, they didn't see her as one of the team's offensive threats anymore. Rather, they wanted her to concentrate on providing leadership to the team.

That was tough for her to hear, as it would have been for anyone. But in retrospect, she appreciated that the coaches were direct with her. She had the option to pout. Instead she embraced her role, and she ended up doing it so well that she was named team captain. "I appreciated that they were being honest with me," she says.

Always try to be direct and authentic when offering criticism. People often talk about the sandwich strategy, which advises managers to "sandwich" negative feedback within compliments. To me, that forces the person offering feedback into an apologetic stance. I don't apologize when I'm offering feedback; I see it as a crucial way to help people achieve optimum performance.

The risk of the sandwich method is that it can send a confusing message. If you pretend you're giving compliments, rather than directly asking for a specific improvement, your feedback may not have the desired effect. That said, I do tend to start a tough conversation—whether it's with my sons or my employees—with some language that establishes how much I value my relationship with them. Then I segue into direct statements that describe the change I'm seeking. And that's how I leave things.

To me, the precise method by which feedback is offered is less important than the identity of the person providing it. Let me explain. I subscribe to Harvard Business School senior fellow Bill George's philosophy of authentic leadership, which proposes that the most important part of being an effective leader is character, in the old-fashioned sense of the term. A person with character is someone who commands respect and loyalty thanks to the way that person conducts him or herself. Being kind. Working hard. Leading confidently, with courage. Making the moral choice.

The best leaders, George writes, are like the best musicians and athletes, because they are "constantly developing themselves to increase self-awareness and improve relationships with others." One of the most important aspects of becoming an authentic leader is developing your emotional intelligence, which in turn requires soliciting feedback from others in your life, listening as that advice is delivered, and then acting on the feedback to correct the issue.

It sounds a little Zen, but one way to ensure that others listen to *your* feedback is to model the behavior you seek in others. Criticism can be tricky. If you set an example by being receptive to criticism, listening to it, and acting on it, then others will be much more likely to be receptive when you're offering your feedback to them.

When you're actually delivering advice, do so in person. Be yourself and speak frankly and directly, without getting emotional or negative. Rather than insulting or demeaning anyone, focus on the change your feedback is intended to create. Chances are the person you're talking to will be grateful for the opportunity to improve.

10

HOW CAN I BEAT A SERIOUS CASE OF PROCRASTINATION?

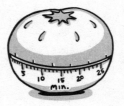

In the mid-1990s, the social psychologists Roy Baumeister and Dianne M. Tice, a married couple who also collaborated in scientific research at Case Western Reserve University in Cleveland, ran a fascinating experiment about procrastination that tested the common adage, "I do my best work under pressure."

Their experiment was designed to test whether procrastination was harmless—or even superior to alternatives. Some procrastinators believe that putting off work until it absolutely has to be done is a technique that brings out superior performance.

To test whether there was any truth to the procrastinators' claims, Tice and Baumeister conducted an experiment on sixty university students. They gave the students an assignment with a deadline near the end of the semester, then told them that they would be able to extend the deadline if they wished. The scientists studied the students as they went through the work cycle, monitoring their health and stress levels and, once they handed in the work, assessing the quality of the submissions.

The diligent workers—those who began work on the project soon after it was first assigned—experienced more stress and illness early in the work cycle. But as the deadline approached, the procrastinators began experiencing more stress and illness, until their stress and poor health surpassed that of the diligent workers. By the end of the semester, the procrastinators suffered far more symptoms of physical illness: eighty-two per week compared with fifty-two for the diligent workers.

And the procrastinators didn't just have more symptoms of ill health; their total stress level was higher than that of the diligent workers.

"Procrastination does not simply shift the same amount of stress and illness from early to late in the project period," Tice and Baumeister wrote. "Rather, it apparently increases the amount of stress and illness."

And after all that, the work the procrastinators handed in wasn't as good, probably because, the researchers speculated, leaving things late had led them to make "compromises and sacrifices in quality." Rather than bringing out the students' best work, delaying the project until near the deadline had elevated their stress, decreased their state of health, and harmed the quality of their work.

So how can one avoid procrastination? It's a question that's increasingly pertinent today, when the incorporation of technology into every aspect of one's life has created a myth of multitasking. My three boys are good at applying themselves to school and handing in assignments on time. They get good grades. I'm not sure I'd be able to be as disciplined as they are amid the pings of text messages and the temptation to check or update umpteen different social media presences.

One useful strategy is the pomodoro technique, developed by an Italian productivity expert named Francesco Cirillo. Its simplest incarnation involves setting a manual, nondigital, ticking kitchen timer to go off in twenty-five minutes and then working hard while the device ticks away. Cirillo calls the twenty-five-minute increment a *pomodoro*, Italian for "tomato," because that was the shape of the timer he used as a university student. Once the twenty-five minutes is up, you take a three- to five-minute break.

I love the idea of the pomodoro because the twenty-five-minute work increment strikes me as just the right duration for a productivity blitz. You're not trying to focus for ten hours straight or working all out until your assignment is done. All you're promising is twenty-five minutes. Even the most die-hard of procrastinators should be able to stave off the temptations of Facebook, Twitter, or the refrigerator for less than half an hour.

Even better is the way Cirillo structures longer durations of working. Essentially, he puts pomodoros together. Before you begin a task, estimate how many pomodoros it will require. Maybe you judge that the task will require three hours. At twenty-five minutes each, that works out to about seven pomodoros.

First, set your physical timer—the lower tech and more tactile, the better. An actual ticking timer is said to help because the ticking is a reminder to maintain your focus. I also find listening to music useful. Promise yourself that for the next twenty-five minutes you will work only on the task at hand. No interruptions. No distractions. Don't let your focus waver, even if another urgent task occurs to you. Keep a paper notepad close at hand, and if a secondary task pops into your mind, write it down, then continue working on your original task.

When the timer rings and the twenty-five minutes is up, get your notepad and put a check mark on the paper beside whatever you've completed—think of it as a little mental reward. Then take a break of a few minutes. Consider walking and standing during your break. (The pomodoro technique syncs up nicely with the latest health research that suggests breaking up long bouts of sitting.) You could get more ambitious with your activity—body-weight squats, jumping jacks, or even push-ups will work. If you can swing it, consider tackling that little task you wrote down while you were focused on building your model. When you're recharged, reset your timer to twenty-five minutes, make your mental oath to focus on a single task, and get to it.

CAN YOU APPLY THE POMODORO TECHNIQUE TO OTHER THINGS THAN WORK?

Absolutely. I think the notion of breaking big things into small pieces is a useful way to manage many different aspects of life. For example, marathons. Back when I was regularly running the 26.2-mile event, I would take short breaks at the water stations situated every few miles throughout the course. The strategy transformed the race from an enormous undertaking to a series of short challenges. I wasn't running an entire marathon; all that I was doing was getting to the next water station. In some ways, life is a marathon. Use the pomodoro technique to get something significant done every day, and you will be amazed at your productivity.

Cirillo suggests taking a longer break every four pomodoros—twenty or thirty minutes is long enough to grab lunch or a quick coffee at your nearby spot. And it's enough time to come back with a fresh and rejuvenated mind for another spate of pomodoros.

Teams can use the pomodoro to focus on a single task during

a meeting. Tackle the unread messages in your email inbox with a pomodoro. Or use one to process the receipts you accumulated during your last business trip. Anything that you find vaguely unpleasant, that you've been putting off, and that has been causing you stress can be dealt with using this strategy.

Remember, according to Tice and Baumeister, if you avoid procrastination, you'll experience better health and less stress—and do higher-quality work in the process.

11

CAN I GET BY ON FIVE HOURS
OF SLEEP A NIGHT?

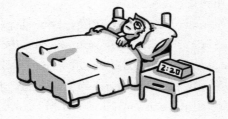

"No" is the short answer. Many workaholics pride themselves on how little sleep they get. It's a badge of honor for them.

In fact, lots of us these days are trying to function on a lot less sleep than we need. The United States has better stats on this than Canada, partly because the US Centers for Disease Control and Prevention has labeled the problem a "public health epidemic." The number of US adults who sleep less than six hours a day nearly doubled from 38.6 million to 70.1 million between 1985 and 2012. The CDC is so concerned that it awarded a grant to two organizations of scientists to study the problem and try to convince people to get more sleep.

What's the problem? Why are people getting so little sleep? Judging from my own family, I have to say that such anytime amusements as television, tablet computers, video games, and phone apps are a large part of the problem.

"We have a lot more distractions than we ever have, even

compared to ten or fifteen years ago," says Dr. Charlene Gamaldo, the medical director of the Johns Hopkins Center for Sleep at How-ard County General Hospital in Columbia, Maryland. "Now we have not only more networks, we have Netflix and the opportunity to binge watch for hours, and the Internet. Plus as high performers we need to stay plugged into our work 24/7. All of these things have happened at the expense of sleep."

One of the most fascinating things about sleep is how little we know about it. For centuries, the common scientific conception was that the brain simply switched itself off when we closed our eyes at night. It wasn't until 1953 that a pair of University of Chicago physi-ologists discovered the existence of cycles in brain activity while we sleep—what would eventually come to be called rapid eye move-ment. Later, Mircea Steriade at Laval University in Quebec discov-ered that brain cells were active in cycles between the REM stages, a phase called slow-wave sleep. Then, in 1994, neurobiologists at an Israeli university established that sleep could improve cognitive performance. Subsequent experiments by other scientists showed that durations of more than six hours were required to trigger this improvement.

Today, we know that sleep plays an important role in the pro-cessing of lived experiences, as well as in learning and retaining in-formation. While our eyes are closed, the brain is sifting through our memories, reliving some of them, weighing what's important and what's not, and making connections between disparate-seeming ex-periences. The brain also returns to problems that stumped us while we were awake. If we want to retain new and complex information or to discover patterns in that information, a good night's sleep is necessary. Essentially, the brain's relationship with information fol-lows a cycle, which the Harvard Medical School physicians and sleep researchers Robert Stickgold and Jeffrey M. Ellenbogen characterize in a *Scientific American Mind* article as "Acquire by day; process by night."

If you don't sleep, the effects add up. Among other things, during nighttime rest, the brain may work to filter out toxic proteins associated with the development of Alzheimer's disease, such as beta-amyloid.

In fact, the less sleep you get and the longer you maintain a sleep deficit, the worse your cognitive performance will turn out to be. "It's like not having enough water to drink," Dr. Gamaldo says. "I can function when I'm thirsty—but I'm not at my best."

To learn the effects of sleep deprivation, one classic experiment limits college students to four or five hours a night for two weeks and then tests their basic cognitive abilities, such as reaction time and attention span. Next, they're allowed to get eight hours of sleep and tested again. "The difference is phenomenal," says Dr. Gamaldo. "Folks who are sleep deprived, even their ability to recover from injury, their immune system response to sickness—it's all impacted even if you get one hour less than your body needs."

One of the most surprising ways that sleep affects overall health, though, may be via body weight. The worldwide expert in metabolism and sleep is Eve Van Cauter, a professor at the University of Chicago, who believes that chronic sleep deprivation is a major factor in the North American obesity epidemic; she speculates that sleep loss may lead to problems with glucose metabolism, which has been associated with greater appetite.

So what's the best amount of sleep for optimum health? That was the question two organizations of scientists joined forces to examine in 2013. Weighing the evidence on numerous different risk factors, the team considered hundreds of different studies and concluded that the minimum duration for maintaining optimum health is seven hours a night.

Different people have different optimum levels of sleep, however—which is one of the reasons the scientists limited their recommendation to a *minimum*. One way to assess how much sleep is optimum for you is to pay attention to how long you stay in bed during a long vacation. If you find by the end of it that you're getting nine hours of sleep a night, you may need the same amount to function at your optimum level when you're back at work.

How can you ensure that you get enough sleep? I'm careful about the amount I get each night. I need what the experts recommended—about seven hours—to feel at my best. As a result, I use routines suggested by the experts to make sure I get a good night's rest.

First, I avoid using backlit tablet computers or phones in the hours before going to bed, because the blue light emitted by the devices prolongs wakefulness. If I wake up in the middle of the night, I stave off the temptation to check my device and concentrate on my breathing, sometimes even counting individual breaths, to avoid anxiety over work and return to sleep quickly.

Many of us know people who take pride in getting by on five hours of sleep a night or even less. I can't help but think that those people would perform better if they were allowing themselves a few more hours in bed. Sleep is a thief, says the old maxim, because it steals half one's life. But that's wrong. In many ways, getting at least seven hours a night promotes a well-lived life.

12

HOW CAN I STAY CALM AND
PERFORM WELL IN A CRISIS?

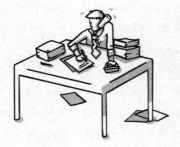

The best way to be certain that you'll stay calm in a crisis is to practice. Simulate the situation beforehand so that when you do encounter a problem, you execute your training.

Curt Cronin encountered crises all the time during the sixteen years he spent as a Navy SEAL, many of them leading teams of his fellow soldiers in the years after the 2001 World Trade Center attacks. For example, say Cronin was leading a team into a dangerous compound and they begin to receive fire. For most people, that would be a major crisis. But not for Cronin; he'd encountered that situation during his training.

"People say you rise to the level of your challenge," he says, "but I believe you fall to the level of your training."

Teams such as the SEALs and Canada's Joint Task Force 2 are masters of preparation. Their missions tend to be rapid deployments. They get in, execute their plan, and get out. One mission might entail parachuting into a compound in Helmand Province with the aim of seizing a computer hard drive that contains the names and details of people who fund terrorism all over the world. From the time the team parachutes from a plane to start the mission to when the Black Hawk helicopters retrieve them from enemy territory, only two hours might have passed. But to prepare for those two hours, they've engaged in dozens, if not hundreds, of hours of preparation. Their days are spent rehearsing contingencies. What happens if we get shot at? What if the hard drive isn't there? What if one of us sustains a debilitating injury?

To illustrate the benefits of preparation, Cronin recalls an incident from early in his SEAL career: the first time he jumped out of an airplane. All that he could see below him was the land, rushing up at him. "I was massively overwhelmed," he recalls. His reaction was characteristic of what happens to most people in a crisis. When we're confronted with a challenge, we tend to fixate on something. "There's so much information to sort through, we're not sure what information to utilize."

The fifth time he jumped out of a plane was different. That time, he was aware of the other people jumping with him. He noticed clouds and the feel of the wind on his face. The twentieth time, he was even more observant. What was the difference? It wasn't that the jump was happening more slowly. Rather, the more times he encountered the same situation, the less he panicked.

"If you're spending time wondering 'How do I respond to this?' then you're at risk," Cronin says. "You're not returning fire. You're not suppressing the threat. You're frozen."

We don't have the time required to run through every conceivable crisis scenario we might face in our business and personal worlds. Nevertheless, problems do happen. And when they're impossible to foresee, preparation is impossible.

To deal with those sorts of scenarios, the elite performance coach Peter Jensen likes to use the example of a sales associate giving a presentation to an important client. The sales associate has prepared her pitch. She's anticipated every question about the product that's imaginable. She's memorized the presentation cold. Moments before the event starts, she sets up in the conference room, connects her laptop to the projector, and launches into her preamble—and then the client holds up his hand. "We're no longer interested in Product A," he announces before everyone. "What can you tell us about Product B?"

Panic is a natural response. As is anger—why didn't the client offer some sort of warning? "Your face gets red, arms cross, you sweat, your pulse is racing," Jensen says. "You have this emotional soup going on."

The danger here, Jensen says, is that the sales associate *becomes* her feelings. She's no longer in charge. Rather, she's a bundle of panic, fear, and disappointment—so much so that she's frozen. She can't react to what's happening.

One possibility is that she fumbles through the rest of the meeting, obviously discombobulated, never taking advantage of the opportunity to sell the client on Product B.

Another possibility? She uses a performance tool Jensen has devised specifically to deal with situations in which practice and preparation are impossible. It comes with an unfortunate acronym—he calls it the FART technique, which stands for "First, ask or repeat the threat."

Asking or repeating the threat is a way to return your mind to an active awareness of what's going on. Another way to think of it is as a way of regaining control of the situation. In the sales meeting, the associate might use the technique to stall for time. "I don't understand where this is coming from," she might say. "Can you help me determine what's changed?"

Sure, it's a stall. But while the client is responding, the associate uses the time to collect herself. To focus on her breathing for a moment. Inhale, exhale. The panic subsides. She grows calmer. And by the time the client stops talking, she's back in charge of herself, ready to adapt to whatever the situation demands.

"No one knows you're doing it," Jensen explains. "But the point is, all of you comes back into the meeting, as opposed to just the part of you that's frightened and panicked. What you're really trying to do is manage what's going on *inside* of you so you can perform better on the outside."

So if you want to perform well in a crisis, first, make like Curt Cronin and the other Navy SEALs, who practice and prepare for every contingency possible. That way, when a crisis does arise, you can respond immediately, rather than spend time thinking about how to deal with it. And if something arises that does throw you for a loop, use Peter Jensen's FART technique to stall for time, regain control of your body and your mind, and then roll with the new situation.

13

HOW SHOULD I WARM UP FOR WORK?

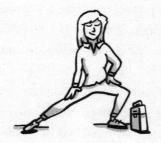

In 2017, at the age of thirty-four, Frenchman Grégory Gaultier became the oldest squash player ever to hold the sport's number one ranking. One of the keys to Gaultier's success is the way he prepares for a big match—a process that bears a lot of similarities to the way people who treat career performance seriously prepare for a big presentation or meeting.

On match day, after he's done all of his physical workouts and strategy discussions, he focuses on one thing: visualization. He goes through what-if scenarios and then imagines the best response. "I close my eyes," he says. "I breathe, relax, and I see myself moving on the court."

Gaultier believes that his visualization preloads his nervous system with reactions. When he is confronted with a problem during the match—such as a ball that falls close to his backhand wall—he doesn't have to stop and think of a solution. The visualization exercises from his warm-up mean he's already thought that scenario through, so he's better able to solve the problem quickly and successfully.

"The visualization makes me react faster," he says.

Squash may not look as though it has a lot of similarities to a business meeting. Gaultier is trying to bounce a little ball around a room, while a typical employee is working through a PowerPoint deck or otherwise managing the meeting. But there are elements of Gaultier's match-day preparation that can apply to business.

"So much of my sport is mental," he says. "Confidence is important. You have to project a certain feeling, because that can influence your opponent."

The highest performers in any field tend to have routines they use to prepare themselves for the occasions that require their greatest performances. The Medcan registered dietitian Rachel Hannah, an elite cross-country runner, also engages in visualization exercises. "It can help to minimize stress," she says.

Brad Stulberg and Steve Magness, the authors of *Peak Performance: Elevate Your Game, Avoid Burnout, and Thrive with the New Science of Success*, refer to this practice as "priming." "Whether it's a writer preparing to draft a story, an athlete prepping for competition, or a businessperson heading into a high-stakes presentation, great performers never just *hope* they'll be on top of their game," they wrote. "Rather, they actively create the specific conditions that will elicit their personal best, priming themselves for performance."

To create your priming routine, first, identify the most important parts of your week. You likely don't have a world championship squash match on the docket, but perhaps you're pitching an investor for seed financing for your start-up. Maybe you're preparing an important brief. Or you have to build something within a limited amount of time. Ask yourself, what can I do to prepare for this job's important events? Work backward from the event itself to the hours before, the days before, the week before. Conduct your research and outline the scenarios.

The most important part of a premeeting "warm-up" is Gaultier's visualization techniques, which I've adopted myself: before an important occasion I'll set aside my phone, close my laptop and my office door, and try to think through every aspect of what's to come.

MUSIC TO MY EARS

The right kind of music can help you warm up for all sorts of occasions. Anyone who has attended a spin class in a studio with a good subwoofer knows that. But music can complement all sorts of situations, particularly today, with wireless speakers, tiny earbuds, and streaming services that offer access to near-infinite libraries of songs for a nominal monthly subscription fee. When I'm walking home from a workout, I'll put my earbuds in to try to maintain the positive endorphins, and then, throughout the day, I'll keep a soundtrack playing while I'm working. The music helps me manage my thoughts and emotions, and it creates a calm environment when I need to concentrate. Silence may be golden, but I find everything a lot more enjoyable with whatever songs my mood favors.

Let's say it's a meeting. I'll visualize myself going in, shaking hands, meeting the various people I'll encounter. I'll think about chitchat and remind myself to maintain my posture. I'll go through potential problems. What if my laptop suddenly dies? The power goes out? Ideally, I've thought through each scenario and come up with a plan for just that occasion—all the way through to the end.

You may not want to conduct an actual physical warm-up before your big meeting—although it's not a bad idea. A brisk walk or some stair climbing can elevate your heart rate and prime your brain for maximum agility. And although I doubt you'll want a protein shake immediately before, you will want to make sure your blood sugar is well regulated, which means eating a meal an hour or two before the meeting's start time.

Finally, standardizing your routine is important. If you have a preparatory series of steps that you can run through, you have something that transitions you from average to elite, a protocol that elevates your awareness from standby to switched on.

One writer friend I know uses visualization techniques to ensure that he's adequately prepared for the two-hour writing block he conducts each morning. A TV presenter uses similar techniques in the moments before she goes on her morning show. The point is, if you want to excel, have a routine that you follow and that makes you feel prepared. Make sure it includes visualization exercises that prime you for every aspect of the scenario ahead. If you want to perform like a champion, you have to warm up like a champion.

14

WHAT'S THE BEST WAY TO
BEAT STAGE FRIGHT?

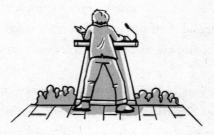

The worst case of stage fright I've faced happened in 2009, before the first True Patriot Love gala dinner that we staged in Toronto. Some of the highest-ranking members of the Canadian military were there, as was then prime minister Stephen Harper. I got up on-stage and looked out at the crowd, and there was a terrible moment where I just blanked. I'd rehearsed my speech so much that I knew it cold, but as I stood there before an audience of 2,000 people, I couldn't have told you the opening few words.

The first thing that people should know about stage fright is that it's enormously common. "What happens," Peter Jensen, the performance coach, says, "is whenever your arousal level goes up, your focus narrows. Whatever the reason—whether you're anxious or you're just overly competitive—it triggers the same mechanism in the body."

The problem with that mechanism is that your focus can narrow so much that you forget everything else. In my case, I forgot my speech while the prime minister looked on. Jensen has dealt with athletes who face similarly dire situations. For example, a basketball player who steps up to the free-throw line and freezes because she's focusing on the crowd. Or a figure skater who forgets her routine moments before she steps onto the ice.

In each case, we begin obsessing about something that distracts us from the task at hand. At one Winter Olympics, Jensen was sitting alongside a female figure skater he'd been coaching. Ten minutes before she was to compete, she turned to Jensen and said, "Peter, I'm really nervous."

Jensen looked at her and saw that she was right. In fact, the young woman was so nervous that her anxiety threatened to prevent her from performing. So Jensen asked, "What else are you?"

At first she didn't know what he meant.

"What kind of shape are you in?" Jensen asked.

The young woman shrugged. "I'm in the best shape of my life."

"What about your program—how's that?"

"My program is great," she said, referring to the routine of axels and toe loops she was about to execute.

"How's your confidence?" Jensen asked.

"My confidence levels have been amazing," she said.

Jensen was trying to get the woman to reframe her thinking. Of course she was anxious—she was about to perform at the Olympics. It was the culminating moment of her young life. It would be a little crazy if she *weren't* nervous. But that wasn't the important thing that would dictate how she would do. What was important was all the other stuff—how she'd practiced, her fitness level, her confidence. So Jensen summed everything up in reverse: "You're in great shape, your program is great, your confidence is great—*and* you're nervous."

Then he asked, "Have you centered?"

Centering is what Jensen calls his breathing exercise. At that first True Patriot Love gala, I would have loved to have had a little Peter Jensen on my shoulder, whispering words of wisdom before I spoke. But when that's not possible, Jensen suggests centering, a breathing exercise he also refers to as *ABC*, for Awareness, Breathing, Choose.

"The minute you focus on your breath," he says, "it shuts down everything else. You're focusing on your diaphragm, the breath entering through the nostrils, and it brings you back to the moment."

So when faced with stage fright or any other form of performance anxiety, the first step is to notice what's happening. In step two, breathe slowly and steadily. Pay attention to every aspect of the respiratory cycle. Inhale, fill the chest, notice how that feels, and exhale. That will direct your focus away from what's threatening to obsess you, whether it's the crowd or the fact that you suddenly can't remember how to shoot a basketball.

In step three, redirect your attention. The initial move to focus on your breathing will calm you down. Once your anxiety is under control, your focus can broaden. Your panic will diminish. It may yet still be there. But you're also focusing on your preparation, your hard work, and your great previous performances in similarly fraught situations.

When world champion figure skater Elvis Stojko stood in his skates at center ice, about to begin a performance, he would conduct Jensen's breathing exercises. Hundreds of other athletes Jensen has advised have done the same in similar moments of intense pressure. When I froze at the beginning of my speech, I thought back to Jensen's ABC. A few breaths in, my panic subsided, a door somewhere in my brain opened, and the words of my speech returned. I still use Jensen's breathing exercises anytime I feel any sort of performance anxiety coming on. I recommend that you do, too.

15

HOW CAN I CULTIVATE A SOCIAL LIFE
WHEN I BARELY HAVE TIME TO WORK?

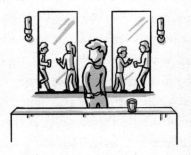

This is a tricky question. We all go through periods when we can't afford the time to think about a social life. One of the reasons that maintaining contact with friends is so difficult is because, like exercise, taking time for such pursuits can make you feel guilty. It can feel self-indulgent. But it's important—especially during challenging periods—to make sure we have strong relationships with our friends and family.

Mitch Prinstein, a University of North Carolina professor of psychology and neuroscience, recently wrote a book about the health effects of social relationships. He cited a fascinating scientific analysis that looked into the link between mortality and the number and quality of people's relationships. It revealed a strong association between our life spans and the quality and complexity of our social lives. As Prinstein wrote in the *New York Times*, the extent to which we feel either socially connected or isolated, disconnected, and lonely can predict how long we'll live—to a remarkable extent.

"Those who had good-quality relationships had a 91 percent higher survival rate," he noted in a *New York Times* article, citing the analysis. "This suggests that being unpopular increases our chance of death more strongly than obesity, physical inactivity or binge drinking. In fact, the only comparable health hazard is smoking."

Prinstein believes the health effects of our social relationships may have something to do with evolution. Early in human development, our capacity for cooperation—working together, say, to hunt and kill prey—dictated whether we lived or died. Seen from this perspective, it makes sense that popularity—that is, the ability to form productive social ties—influences human longevity today. Years ago, solo humans tended to die earlier because they were more susceptible to ambush by other predators. Today, those same solo humans still tend to die earlier, but now the cause is related to loneliness.

It's not just being popular that matters, though—the *type* of popularity is important, too. Your life span isn't just dictated by the number of social connections you have. What influences human happiness, success, and health is likability, or, as Prinstein describes it, "kindness, benevolent leadership and selfless, prosocial behavior."

But how can you maintain a social life amid so many competing demands for your time? I think it helps to cut yourself some slack in this department. We have to accept that there are going to be periods in our lives when we're just too busy to make socializing a priority—when your kids are young, for example, or when you're building your career.

Things will inevitably change: kids grow up; careers stabilize. And along the way, there are strategies to manage your social life so that it doesn't take as much time as you may think.

To start, consider combining different aspects of your life:

exercise, social, and work. You might start a fitness group with work colleagues, for example. Or head to a museum with your family.

Tim Hockey, the CEO of TD Ameritrade, established a cycling group designed for business leaders to go riding together. They called themselves Les Domestiques—the servants—because another of their efforts is philanthropy. Today they number several dozen. In a decade, they've raised more than a quarter of a billion dollars for local charities. The group has also had a major impact on Hockey's social life. He says he now relies on the group for the majority of his non-family-related socializing.

"You're the average of the people you hang around with," he says. "So you have to choose your friends wisely."

Most of us aren't able to found a social group devoted to philanthropic causes. But social contact is important for everyone, and many of us can learn from Hockey's template of combining social relationships with other parts of one's life. Creating exercise appointments with friends is one way. Founding a sports team and populating it with your favorite people is another. If you feel so overwhelmed by work and family demands that you can't imagine carving out enough time to catch up with friends and family separately, consider combining several aspects of your life.

HOW CAN I MAINTAIN A MENTAL
EDGE AS I GROW OLD?

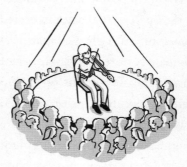

One of the more brilliant figures in the field of aging research is the Northwestern University medical school professor Marsel Mesulam. In a 2013 study, he noted the widespread belief that "a gradual loss of intellectual ability is part of 'normal' aging." But then he made a happy observation: "It turns out that this disarmingly simple assumption is extremely difficult to substantiate or refute."

In other words, according to Mesulam, it's difficult to prove that one of the key things we associate with growing older—a gradual decline in cognitive function—is actually tied to the passage of time. The idea that our brains inevitably and irreparably decline may not be so true after all.

In 1994, researchers performed cognitive tests on a thousand medical doctors ranging in age from 28 to 92 years old. Those who were younger than 35 achieved an average score that was much higher than those who were older than 75. But then the researchers looked at the top performers in each category. They were shocked to discover that the scores of the ten best subjects under the age of 35 were about the same as the ten best subjects over the age of 75.

So it's clearly possible to retain your faculties as you age. Mesulam calls the people who do so *SuperAgers*. How do SuperAgers resist the mental decline that we associate with aging? Mesulam and his team studied a cohort of people who exhibited superior cognitive performance past the age of 80. They discovered that the cerebral cortex in SuperAgers' brains is thicker than average. Also, Super-Agers' anterior cingulate cortexes contain fewer Alzheimer's disease–associated protein tangles. The brains of SuperAgers also tend to contain much higher concentrations of von Economo neurons, a type of nerve cell associated with greater intellectual capacity.

All of that brings us to the most relevant question: How can one become a SuperAger? Scientists do not yet have conclusive proof. It may be possible that superaging is exclusively genetic. But the evidence suggests that certain lifestyle choices may help to preserve memory. The activities that light up the superaging centers of the brain tend to be things that require hard work—whether that work is physical or mental.

In an article written for the *New York Times*, psychology professor Lisa Feldman Barrett, who has conducted important research on SuperAgers, suggested that a pleasant round of after-dinner Sudoku isn't hard enough. "You must expend enough effort that you feel some 'yuck.' Do it until it hurts, and then a bit more," she wrote. ". . . if people consistently sidestep the discomfort of mental effort or physical exertion, this restraint can be detrimental to the brain. . . . If you don't use it, you lose it."

Here, then, are five strategies that may help you become a SuperAger—with some suggestions on ways to apply pressure in a manner that amps up the mental exertion.

MASTER A MUSICAL INSTRUMENT AND
THEN STAGE A PUBLIC PERFORMANCE

Pleasant, once-weekly lessons may not tax the brain enough. Rather, sign up to participate in a recital or arrange an upcoming solo at a pub night, and then pledge to do your best.

TAKE A FOREIGN LANGUAGE COURSE
THAT REQUIRES A FINAL EXAM

It may not be enough to simply enroll in a continuing education class at your local university. Try to ensure that your coursework is rigorous enough to require prolonged study, and set a goal to prove something to the younger students by getting the top marks in the concluding exam.

PLAY CONTRACT BRIDGE IN TOURNAMENTS

It's not a coincidence that people such as Bill Gates and Warren Buffett are fanatics for bridge. The card game requires lots of strategic calculation, and regular participation in the numerous tournament events that occur every year is a great way to force the brain to perform mental gymnastics.

COACH A YOUTH SPORTS TEAM

Amateur athletics organizations—whether soccer, hockey, figure skating, swimming, or other sport—can always use knowledgeable volunteers. Join one, and study up on the tactics required for your club to ensure excellence at competitive events. Don't let those kids down!

CONTINUE TO WORK AT YOUR
BRAIN-DEMANDING JOB

If your work features pressure and thinking, sidestep retirement for as long as possible and try to put the emphasis on projects that require developing new bodies of knowledge or forms of thinking.

Maintaining a mental edge requires hard work. To stay sharp, you have to put yourself into situations that tax your brain. No one looks forward to having their mental faculties decline. Most of us know that exercising the body hard will stave off physical decline. It turns out that the same may be true for our mental capabilities. What's good for the body is also good for the mind.

ACKNOWLEDGMENTS

First of all, I want to recognize two different groups that inspire me every day. The clients of Medcan and EHE are the best wellness partners around. Their stories inspire my own life and shape the way we provide our services. I feel lucky to be able to work with them.

The military families I've encountered as the chair of True Patriot Love and an organizer of the 2017 Invictus Games, and especially on the expeditions to such locations as the Himalayas and the Canadian Arctic, are frequently in my thoughts. Their sacrifice sets an example I admire and hope to live up to.

I've long known that a book is a communal effort, the product of the labor of a whole community of interested people. But now that this one is done, I feel I have a new understanding of the truth of that statement. This book could not have been written without the generosity and knowledge of more than a hundred topic experts who contributed their time and, more important, their opinions on dozens of different wellness issues. Their names are too many to mention here. Suffice it to say, if you're quoted as an expert within this book, I am grateful.

Dr. Michael Parkinson provided the phrase that eventually became this title. I'm grateful to him for allowing me to use it.

The various professional staff who worked on this book have impressed me with their dedication to its success. At Simon & Schuster, I'm grateful to director of publicity and Canadian sales, Adria Iwasutiak. Brendan May was the editor whose intelligence and wisdom elevated every aspect of this book. Simon & Schuster publisher Kevin Hanson runs a tight ship. My agent, Michael Levine, believed in this book from the beginning, got it sold, and entertained me every step of the way with his wealth of Canadian media anecdotes. And in my second decade of working with my writing collaborator, Christopher Shulgan, I remain impressed with his ability to construct compelling and readable prose out of our entertaining discussions.

Numerous smart people went over various drafts of the book. Their suggestions made the book more compelling, more factually accurate, and, in general, better in every way. I'm grateful in particular to the Medcan team of registered dietitians for their help on the Eat section: Leslie Beck, Alex Friel, Stefania Palmeri, Vandana Gujadhur, and Rachel Hannah. The Move section was compiled with the help of Carrie Siu Butt and trainers Chris Campbell, Chris Mear, and Timothy Evangelista. Mike Friedman contributed his advice and expertise in the Think section.

The employees of both Medcan and EHE inspire me every day with their dedication to the cause of promoting wellness among our clients. Thanks to all my colleagues for helping make this book a success.

Thank you to my trainer, Thomas Adriaens, for keeping me fit. And to my assistant, Kate Kulcheski, for keeping my life on track.

My family improves my life in ways too numerous to count.

Thanks to my father, Dr. Robert Francis, who founded Medcan in 1987 and believed in my ability to bring it to the next level. My mother, Sharon, was a key part of Medcan's success in the early years and selflessly made many sacrifices that set up my father and her children with the opportunities we had.

My children, RJ, William, and Christopher, have deepened my appreciation for life. Most of all, thank you to my wife, Stacy, who sets an example for excellence that I aspire to match.